Diverticular Disease: Emerging Evidence in a Common Condition

FALK SYMPOSIUM 148

Diverticular Disease: Emerging Evidence in a Common Condition

Edited by

W. Kruis
Evangelical Hospital
Cologne
Germany

A. Forbes
University College Hospital
London
UK

K.-W. Jauch
University Clinic Munich
Munich
Germany

M.E. Kreis
University Clinic Munich
Munich
Germany

S.D. Wexner
Cleveland Clinic Florida
Weston, FL
USA

Proceedings of the Falk Symposium 148 held in Munich, Germany, June 17–18, 2005

Springer

Library of Congress Cataloging-in-Publication Data is available.

ISBN-10 1-4020-4317-1
ISBN-13 978-14020-4317-8

Published by Springer,
PO Box 17, 3300 AA Dordrecht, The Netherlands

Sold and distributed in North, Central and South America
by Springer,
101 Philip Drive, Norwell, MA 02061 USA

In all other countries, sold and distributed
by Springer,
PO Box 322, 3300 AH Dordrecht, The Netherlands

Printed on acid-free paper

Contents

List of principal contributors

WH Aldoori
Wyeth Consumer Healthcare Inc
5975 Whittle Road
Mississauga
Ontario, L4Z 3M6
Canada

S Bar-Meir
Chaim Sheba Medical Center
Department of Gastroenterology
2 Sheba Road
52 621 Tel Hashomer
Israel

B Egger
Department of Visceral and Transplantation Surgery
Inselspital, University of Bern
CH-3010 Bern
Switzerland

S Feuerbach
Institut für Röntgendiagnostik
Universitätsklinkum Regensburg
Franz-Josef-Strauss-Allee 11
D-93042 Regensburg
Germany

A Fingerhut
Centre Hospitalier Intercommunal
F-78303 Poissy
France

A Forbes
Department of Gastroenterology
University College Hospital
235 Euston Road
London NW1 2BU
UK

S Gasche
Medical University of Vienna
Klinik für Innere Medizin IV
Währinger Gürtel 18-20
A-1090 Vienna
Austria

V Gross
Innere Medizin II
Klinikum St. Marien Amberg
Mariahilfbergweg 7
D-92224 Amberg
Germany

NY Haboubi
Trafford General Hospital
Surgical Pathology
Moorside Road
Davyhulme, Manchester
M41 5SL
UK

JC Hoffmann
Medizinische Klinik I
Charité Universitätsmedizin
Campus Benjamin Franklin (CBF)
Hindenburgdamm 30
D-12200 Berlin
Germany

S Hollerbach
Klinik für Gastroenterologie
Allgemeines Krankenhaus Celle
Siemensplatz 4
D-29223 Celle
Germany

KW Jauch
Klinikum der Universität
München-Grosshadern
Marchioninistrasse 15
D-81377 München
Germany

RH Jones
Department of General Practice and Primary Care
King's College London
5 Lambeth Walk
London, SE11 6SP
UK

H-J Krammer
Department of Medicine II
University Hospital of Heidelberg at Mannheim
Theodor-Kutzer-Ufer 1-3
D-68165 Mannheim
Germany

ME Kreis
Ludwig-Maximilians Universität
Klinikum Grosshadern
Chirurgische Klinik
Marchioninistrasse 15
D-81377 München
Germany

G Latella
Department of Internal Medicine
Gastroenterology Unit
University of L'Aquila
Piazza Salvatore Tommasi 1
I-67100 L'Aquila
Italy

B Lembcke
Medizinische Klinik
St. Barbara-Hospital
Barbarastr. 1
D-45964 Gladbeck
Germany

J Lindsay
St Bartholomew's and the Royal London Hospitals
Barts and the London NHS Trust
Whitechapel
London, E1 1BB
UK

D Meyer
University of Würzburg
Department of Surgery (ZOM)
Oberdurrbacher Strasse 6
D-97080 Würzburg
Germany

MZ Panos
Euroclinic
9 Athanasiadou Street
11 521 Athens
Greece

S Schanz
Department of Internal Medicine and Gastroenterology
Evangelisches Krankenhaus Kalk
Buchforststr. 2
D-51103 Köln
Germany

J Schölmerich
Klinik und Poliklinik für Innere Medizin I
Klinikum der Universität Regensburg
D-93042 Regensburg
Germany

RC Spiller
University Hospital
Queen's Medical Centre
Division of Gastroenterology
C Floor, South Block
Nottingham, NG7 2UH
UK

T Wedel
Institute of Anatomy
University of Lubeck
Ratzeburger Allee 160
D-23538 Lubeck
Germany

List of chairpersons

M Anthuber
Allgemeinchirurgie
Klinikum Augsburg
Stenglinstr. 2
D-86156 Augsburg
Germany

WE Fleig
Innere Medizin I
Martin-Luther-Universität
Halle-Wittenberg
Ernst-Grube-Strasse 40
D-06120 Halle
Germany

C Folwaczny
Klinikum der Universität
München-Innenstadt
Medizinische Poliklinik
Nussbaumstr. 20
D-80336 München
Germany

C Hüscher
Department of Surgery
San Giovanni Hospital
I-00184 Rome
Italy

H Koop
Innere Medizin II
Helios Klinikum Berlin
Klinikum Buch
Hobrechtsfelder Chaussee 100
D-13125 Berlin
Germany

W Kruis
Evang. Krankenhaus Kalk
Innere Medizin
Buchforststr. 2
D-51103 Köln
Germany

P Layer
Innere Medizin
Israelitisches Krankenhaus
Orchideenstieg 14
D-22297 Hamburg
Germany

M Lukas
Charles University
First Faculty of Medicine
V Medical Department
U nemocnice 2
CZ-12808 Praha
Czech Republic

P Marteau
Hôpital Europeen
Georges Pompidou
Service d'Hepato-Gastroenterologie
20, rue Leblanc
F-75908 Paris
France

J Mössner
Innere Medizin II
Universitätsklinikum Leipzig
Philipp-Rosenthal-Strasse 27
D-04103 Leipzig
Germany

D Örtli
Mittlere Strasse 91
CH-4012 Basel
Switzerland

S Post
Chirurgie
Klinikum Mannheim
Theodor-Kutzer-Ufer 1–3
D-68167 Mannheim
Germany

A Revhaug
Department of Surgery
Tromso University Hospital
N-9038 Tromso
Norway

RC Spiller
University Hospital
Queen's Medical Centre
Division of Gastroenterology
C Floor, South Block
Nottingham, NG7 2UH
UK

M Starlinger
Allgemeine Öffentliche
Krankenanstalten
Chirurgische Abteilung
St-Veiter-Strasse 47
A-9026 Klagenfurt
Austria

SD Wexner
Cleveland Clinic Florida
2950 Cleveland Clinic Boulevard
Weston, FL 33331
USA

M Zeitz
Medizinische Klinik I
Charité Universitätsmedizin
Campus Benjamin Franklin (CBF)
Hindenburgdamm 30
D-12203 Berlin
Germany

H Zirngibl
Chirurgie
Helios Klinikum Wuppertal
Heusnerstrasse 40
D-42283 Wuppertal
Germany

Preface

Colonic diverticula are a common finding. In contrast, the number of original contributions to the current literature covering this area is rather sparse. This may have several reasons, either a paucity of open questions or a lack of scientific activity.

Indeed, when discussing diagnosis and treatment of diverticular disease, many unclear details arise. Already definition is disputable. The appropriate diagnostic work-up – in primary or secondary settings or in emergency cases – can be debated and evidence-based recommendations on medical treatment are hardly available. Beyond clinical matters many scientific questions need to be clarified.

Thus, for the first time the idea was born to organize a symposium exclusively focused on diverticular disease of the colon. An unrestricted grant of the Falk Foundation made the plan possible. Thanks to the outstanding hospitality of the Falk family, experts from all over the world were able to bring together current knowledge. The present proceedings are a unique description of a common condition with emerging evidence. It is hoped that the Falk Symposium No. 148 will help to stimulate further clinical and basic research in an area which seems sometimes a little apart from popular topics but which is very important for daily practice.

On behalf of the editorial board
Wolfgang Kruis

Section I
Pathogenesis of diverticular disease

Chair: W. KRUIS and A. REVHAUG

1
Patterns of colonic mucosal inflammation in diverticular disease

N. Y. HABOUBI, A. KHATTAB and M. W. EDILBE

INTRODUCTION

The aim of this chapter is to draw attention to a relatively ill-recognized and ill-understood, as well as rarely documented, condition that affects the luminal aspect of the sigmoid colon in patients with diverticular disease, and in which there are some endoscopic, clinical and pathological changes which may warrant its recognition as a separate entity. On reviewing the literature it appears that the condition probably represents a single entity but with a wide range of clinical, histological and endoscopic features.

We are for the first time proposing a histological classification for diverticular colitis (DC).

DEFINITION AND TERMINOLOGY

Diverticular colitis is best defined as an inflammatory condition, with a wide spectrum of colonoscopic changes and confirmed by microscopic examination. The disease affects the luminal mucosa of the segment of the colon, most frequently the sigmoid, that is affected by diverticular disease (Figure 1).

This inflammatory process is independent of the presence or absence of diverticulitis, i.e. inflammation of the diverticular pouch. These mucosal changes may antedate the emergence of diverticular pouches; that is, they may appear in the prediverticular phase, which is characterized by muscular thickening.

The condition suffers from many synonyms, e.g. segmental colitis[1], crescentic colitis, crescentic mucosal fold[2], sigmoid colitis, sigmoiditis and sigmoid colitis-associated diverticular disease (SCADD).

In this chapter we will use the term diverticular colitis (DC) throughout.

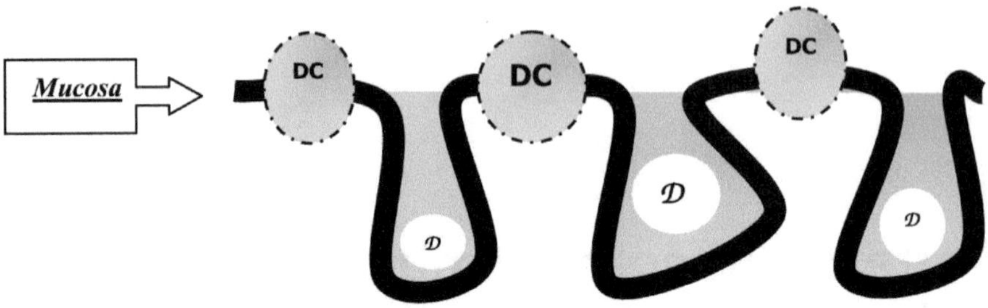

Figure 1 Representation of the diverticulae (D) and the colonic luminal mucosa which is affected by diverticular colitis

PREVALENCE

The exact prevalence of DC has not yet been established, for a variety of reasons. First, there is no general acceptance of DC as a separate condition by pathologists, endoscopists, gastroenterologists or colorectal surgeons. Secondly, the condition is not often presented as an entity, as symptoms can be masked by the associated diverticulitis and the symptoms are often subclinical. Thirdly, some of the cases reported in the literature have subsequently been labelled as ulcerative colitis. This may mean that there is an overlap between the two separate entities, that one of them is common, or simply that DC is not a separate entity and is simply another manifestation of distal ulcerative colitis.

There are few studies addressing the prevalence of DC. Gore et al., in their study of 2380 colonoscopy and sigmoidoscopy episodes collected during a 5-year period, showed that there were mucosal changes in 34 cases (1.42%)[2] only. Another study revealed two cases of chronic colitis out of 151 resected colon cases for diverticulitis[3].

In spite of the huge prevalence of diverticular disease the frequency of DC is extremely low, and there are only 98 cases reported as representing DC in the recent literature[4].

PATHOGENESIS

Although the pathogenesis of DC is not clear, there are undoubtedly many factors contributing to the disease process. These factors can be summarized as follows:

1. The relative shortening of the bowel that occurred in diverticular disease is well described[5]. This bowel shortening leads to mucosal redundancy with subsequent prolapse of the redundant mucosa. These changes may occur in prediverticular disease where there is already abnormal thickening of

muscle, and before the physical creation of diverticula[6,7]. This suggests that intramural and intraluminal changes are more important in the pathogenesis of DC than inflammation of the diverticula themselves, i.e. diverticulitis.

2. Other factors – such as bacterial overgrowth, mucolysis, increased exposure to intraluminal toxins and antigens secondary to faecal stasis and relative ischaemia of mucosa – have all been implicated as important factors in the genesis of DC[8]; moreover, anatomical factors, exposure to intraluminal irritants and trauma have been implicated as reasons for the selective distribution of the inflammatory process in DC[2]. The combination of mucosal prolapse and ischaemia or trauma may contribute to the pathogenesis of cap polyp, which is one of the histological features that characterize DC.

CLINICAL PICTURE

In one study the median age for DC is 72 years, with a range from 38 to 87 years and no noticeable sex differences[3]. In another study DC affects younger patients with a mean age of 60.4 (range 32–87) and a male predominance with male to female ratio of 2.4:1[2].

The clinical presentation is highly variable and patients can present with a range of symptoms[8]. Intermittent rectal bleeding is the most common presentation (83%), but non-localized abdominal pain, tenesmus, chronic constipation, and episodic diarrhoea have all been reported[3]. Some patients suffer from excessive flatulence, vomiting, weight loss and fever[9]. In one study the duration of symptoms ranged from 1 week to several years[3]. Usually there are no external physical signs, although occasionally anaemia and deep left iliac fossa tenderness are reported[10].

DIAGNOSIS

It is important to differentiate DC from other types of sigmoid colitis; these include ischaemic colitis, infective colitis, diverticulitis, inflammatory bowel disease and NSAID-induced colitis[10].

Laboratory findings

These are usually normal, the acute-phase reactants and/or white cell count being increased very rarely[11,12]. Although there are no data on the prevalence of perinuclear antineutrophil cytoplasmic antibody (pANCA) in patients with diverticular colitis, its presence is likely to favour a diagnosis of inflammatory bowel disease, particularly ulcerative colitis[10] (pANCA is found in 70% of patients with ulcerative colitis, in 15% of patients with Crohn's disease and in less than 5% in the general population[13]). In acute presentations stool should be sent for microscopy and culture to rule out infective colitis[10].

The barium enema

This shows the presence of sigmoid diverticula with or without non-obstructing sigmoid stenosis and without specific features[3]. If Crohn's disease is strongly suspected barium follow-through is recommended to inspect the small bowel proximal to the reach of the colonoscope[10].

Ileocolonoscopy

Ileocolonoscopy is needed with biopsies taken from the terminal ileum to detect small bowel Crohn's disease and from the remainder of the colon, especially from the rectum, to exclude, as far as possible, ulcerative colitis[10].

ENDOSCOPIC FINDINGS OF DC

The endoscopic appearances are variable and the only consistent feature is that the luminal inflammation is always confined to the segment of the bowel affected by diverticular disease (i.e. the sigmoid colon and distal descending colon), and often away from the diverticular orifices[2,3,9,8]. The extent of the segment of colon harbouring the endoscopic abnormality varies from 5 to 25 cm[3].

The endoscopic findings range from mild, non-specific changes to florid, active inflammatory changes, and there are always signs of mucosal hyperaemia, granularity, friability or even frank intramucosal haemorrhages[3,4]. Occasionally shallow mucosal depressions without sharp demarcation from the surrounding mucosa have been reported, yet aphthous or linear ulcerations were not observed[3].

These changes may have diffuse distribution[3], irregular patchy distribution discontinuous with diverticular ostia[9] or occasionally the abnormality is circumferentially encompassing diverticular ostia, together with adjacent contiguous mucosa[3].

In crescentic fold disease the mucosal swelling, erythema and haemorrhage are strictly confined to the crescentic mucosal folds with sparing of the diverticular orifices[2]. The patches measure at least 10 mm in diameter[2,9]. The polypoidal prolapse lesion may have an alarming endoscopic appearance, which to the inexperienced endoscopist may suggest a neoplastic process (Figure 2).

PATHOLOGY

The evidence of histological features in DC are prominent mucosal folds, variable degree of lympho-plasmacytic and neutrophils infiltrate into lamina propria, intra-epithelial lymphocytes, granulomas, fibrosis of lamina propria, mucosal ulceration, and variable degree of crypt branching, shortening and dilation[7]. However, broadly speaking, we may see three patterns of microscopic changes in DC; these are categorized as follows:

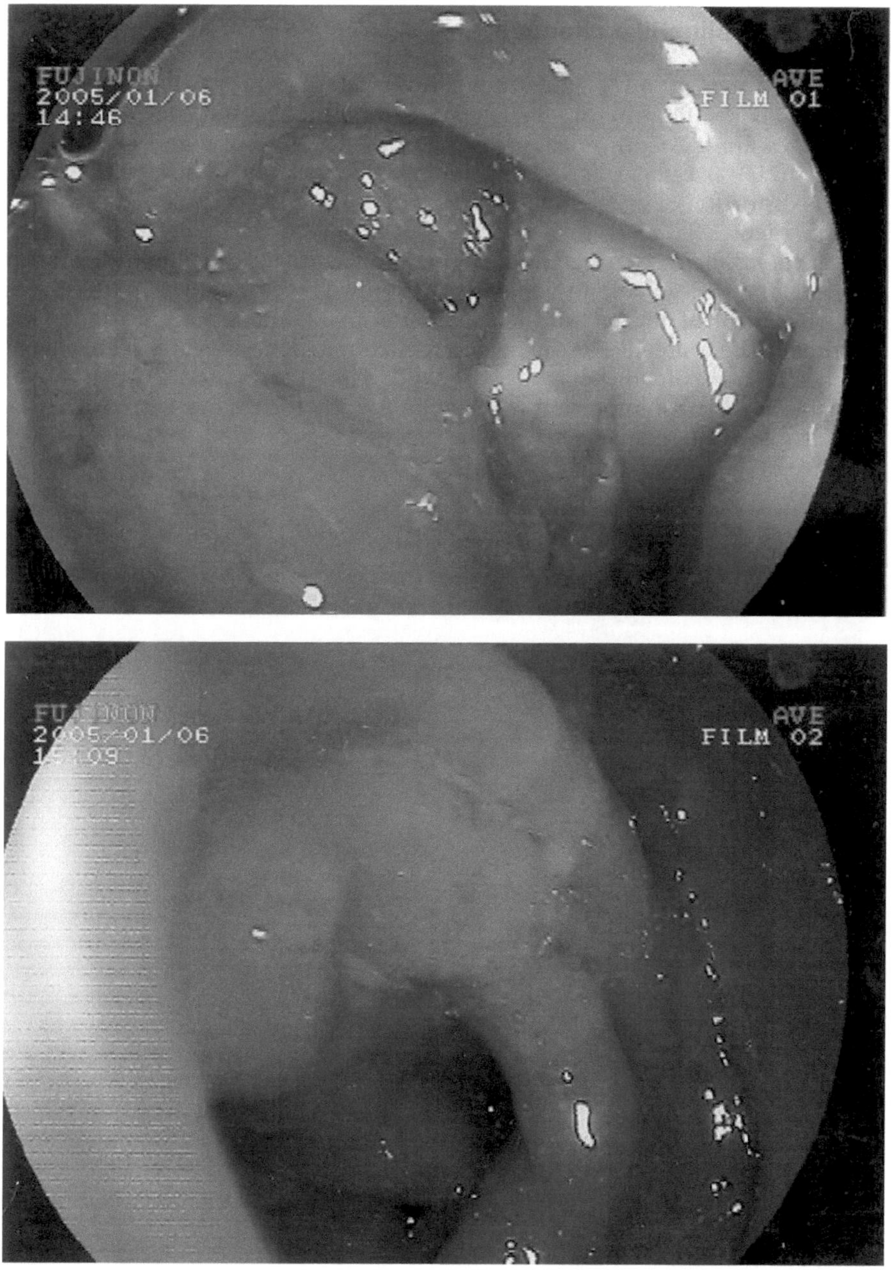

A

B

Figure 2 A case of polypoidal mucosal prolapse in a patient with diverticular disease

Ulcerative colitis-like changes

The Makapugay and Dean study[3] revealed that cryptitis, increase of mononuclear inflammatory cells in lamina propria and basal lymphoid aggregates are the main microscopic findings. These were found in all of the 23 cases (100%). Other microscopic findings were prominent but less common, such as distortion of crypt architecture 20 (87%) and Paneth cell metaplasia 11 (48%)[3] (Figures 3 and 4).

It is very difficult to differentiate between ulcerative colitis and diverticular colitis on the basis of colonoscopic biopsies only. Therefore other findings, such as involvement of the rectum and extension of inflammation into the colon proximally, undoubtedly aid its accurate identification, as rectal involvement practically rules out the diagnosis of DC[4]. This information often becomes available in the most important regular clinicopathological meetings, where the final diagnosis can be reached.

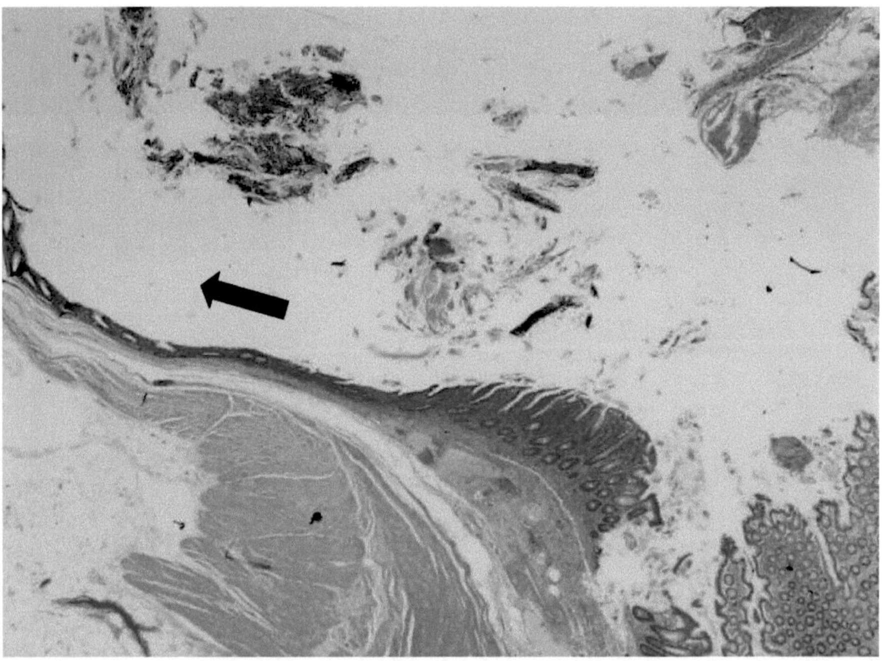

Figure 3 A small focus of diverticular colitis with opening of the mouth of diverticular pouch (arrow)

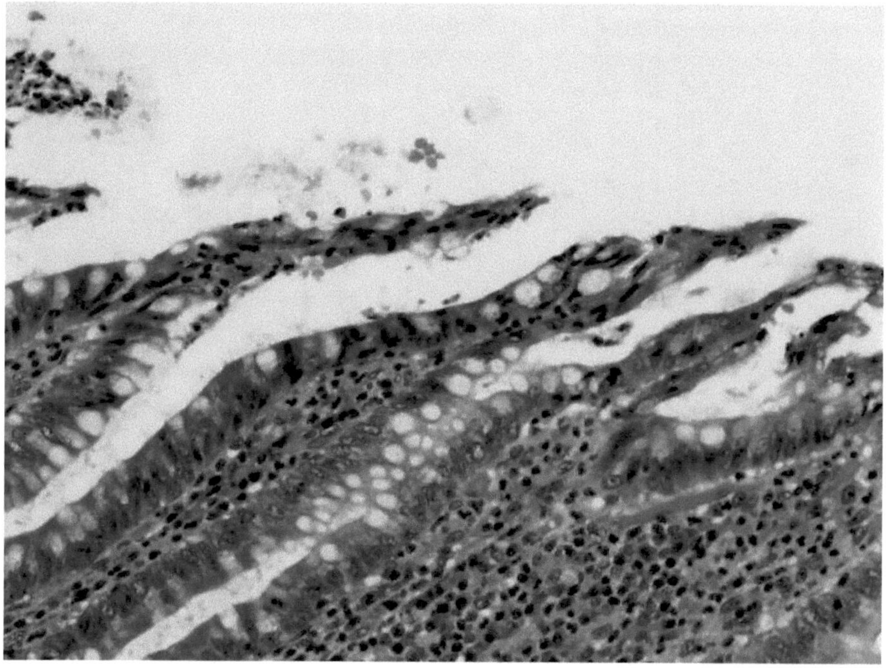

Figure 4 A case of diverticular colitis showing dense, mixed inflammatory cell infiltrate and papillary formation of mucosa is a typical histological picture of chronic colitis

Crohn's disease-like changes

Crohn's disease by and large is strictly a clinicopathological condition, but has certain histological features which, if present and in the background of inflammatory bowel disease, become diagnostic. The most common of these features are non-caseating sarcoid-type granulomas, transmural inflammation, focal mucosal involvement and fissuring ulcerations. Relying on the clinical outcome, the literature is divided as to whether Crohn's-type features are found in cases of DC or simply whether the two conditions coexist. The consensus is in favour of the former proposal. The Meyers et al. study showed that 10 out of 21 cases of diverticulosis had sigmoid granulomatous colitis[5]. The microscopic features for this pattern closely mimicked the changes seen in ordinary Crohn's disease. Characteristic non-caseating granulomas were also found in 17 out of 21 cases of resected colon for diverticulosis, and in the regional lymph nodes in six of the cases, whereas deep fissuring ulcers were remarkable in three of the cases[5]. On the other hand, Goldstein et al. in their study had 24 cases with numerous non-necrotizing granulomas in all the layers of the bowel wall out of 29 resected specimens[7]. Moreover granulomas were not only detected in the mucosa and submucosa of the diverticula, but they were also involved in the wall of the pericolonic adipose tissue and lymph nodes (Figure 5).

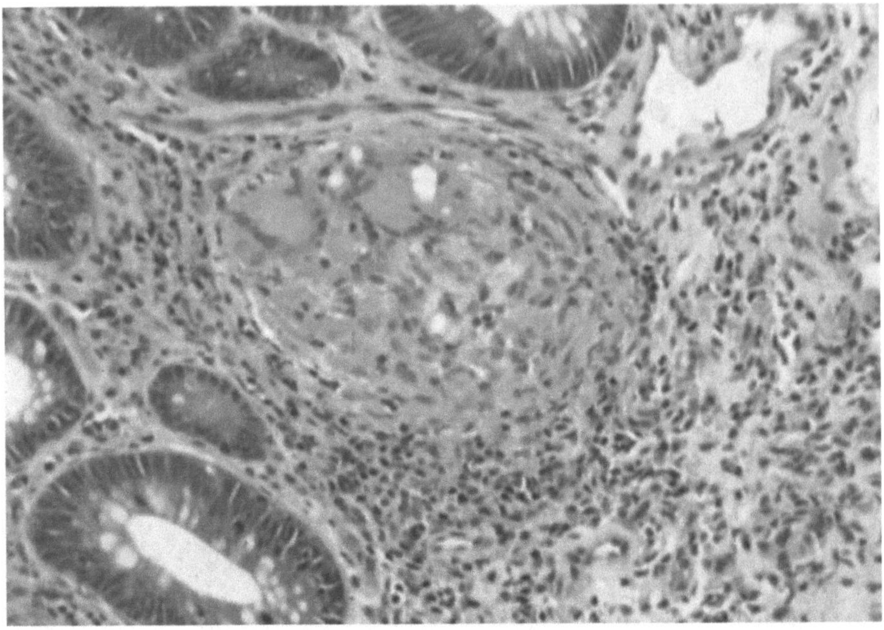

Figure 5 A focus of sarcoid-type granuloma in a case of diverticular colitis

Gledhill and Dixon reported 11 cases of Crohn's disease type-diverticulitis with typical 'classic' histological features of Crohn's disease- like, transmural inflammation, granulomas and ulceration. In nine patients the features were confined to the resected specimens only, and none of these patients progressed to full-blown Crohn's disease[14]. Their conclusion is that the histological changes representing Crohn's disease are reaction processes to diverticulosis rather than to Crohn's disease *per se*. It is important to note that in the early literature some of the cases did develop a full clinical picture of Crohn's disease, but this is at variance with current beliefs. We believe that some cases of diverticular disease may show histological features akin to Crohn's disease, but should not be regarded as Crohn's cases.

In summary, it is important to realize that focal active inflammation, abnormal crypt architecture and granulomas are features that could be found in a few cases of diverticular colitis[2].

Prominent mucosal folds

Prominent mucosal folds are defined as expansion of the fold more than 5 mm above the inner aspect of the muscularis propria. This distance was measured in a particular way by using a ruler placed on the stage, ×2 stage and ×10 eyepiece objective[7] (Figure 6). Goldstein and Ahmad found the prominent mucosal folds were seen in 91 out of 100 sigmoid colon resection specimens

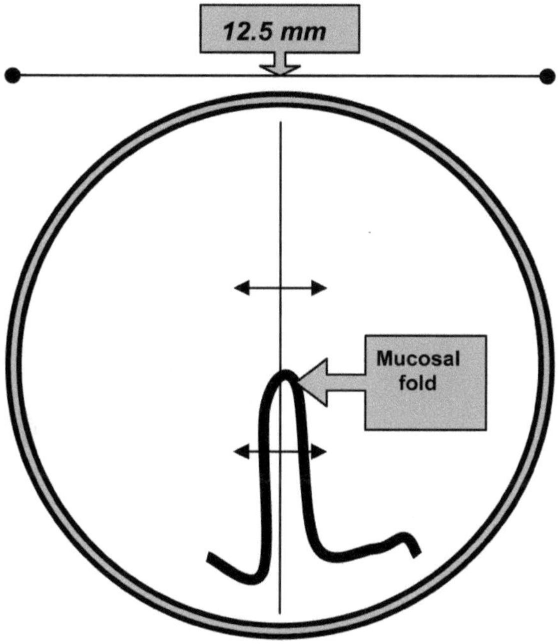

Figure 6 Dimensions of colonic mucosal fold under the microscope using ×2 stage and ×10 eyepiece objective

removed for diverticulitis[7], whereas these changes were noticed in three out of 34 cases in another study[2]. In a further study of eight cases of surgically resected sigmoid colons with diverticular disease, contained protruding mucosal folds or polyps numbered from one to 11 per specimen, ranging from 0.5 to 3.0 cm in greatest dimension[15] (Figure 7). The histological features of the mucosal folds are characterized by polypoidal protrusion of the mucosa which shows an assortment of acute and chronic inflammatory cell infiltrate, fibrosis of lamina propria, crypt distortion and formation of teardrop or diamond-shaped crypts and sometimes proliferation of the muscularis mucosa.

Two special forms may be seen: cap polyp and polypoidal mucosal prolapse (myoglandular polyp). The cap polyp is characterized by ulceration of the luminal part of the polyp and replacement by a variably thick layer of a 'cap' made up of acute inflammatory cells and fibrin (Figure 8). The myoglandular polyp has features similar to solitary ulcer (mucosal herniation syndrome) (Figure 9).

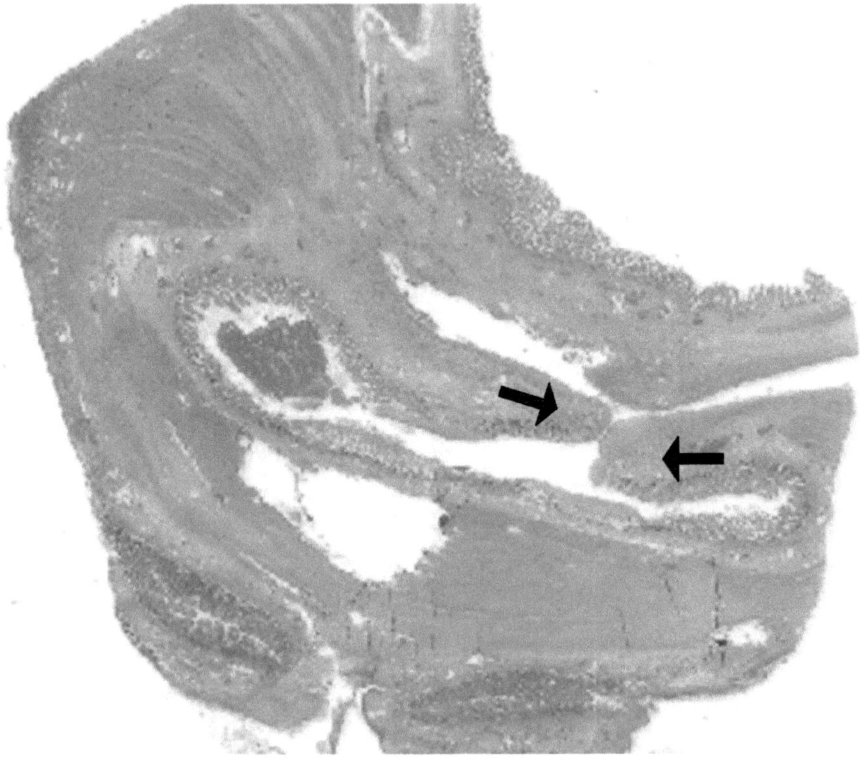

Figure 7 A cross-section of diverticular disease showing polypoidal mucosal herniation (arrows)

TREATMENT

About 50% of patients diagnosed with DC will require some form of therapy to alleviate their symptoms, while the other half will settle spontaneously[2].

A short course of antibiotic, and instructions to increase dietary fibre content, will lead to a symptomatic improvement; that is, cessation of bleeding and resolution of abdominal pain, in approximately 60% of the cases[3]. Therefore, inflammatory bowel disease-directed therapy does not seem to be a mandatory first-line therapeutic option[3]. However, it should be remembered that the elastosis of established diverticular disease is irreversible, and an improvement in diet will have only limited results[4]. In addition to that the use of NSAID should be avoided[10].

Those patients who fail to respond to the above-mentioned treatment will require sulphasalazine or 5-aminosalicylic acid (5-ASA) with or without hydrocortisone or mesalazine enema[2,3,9,16]. In the vast majority of cases sulphasalazine will lead to complete remission within 6 weeks, and the hydrocortisone or mesalazine enema will lead to complete eradication of

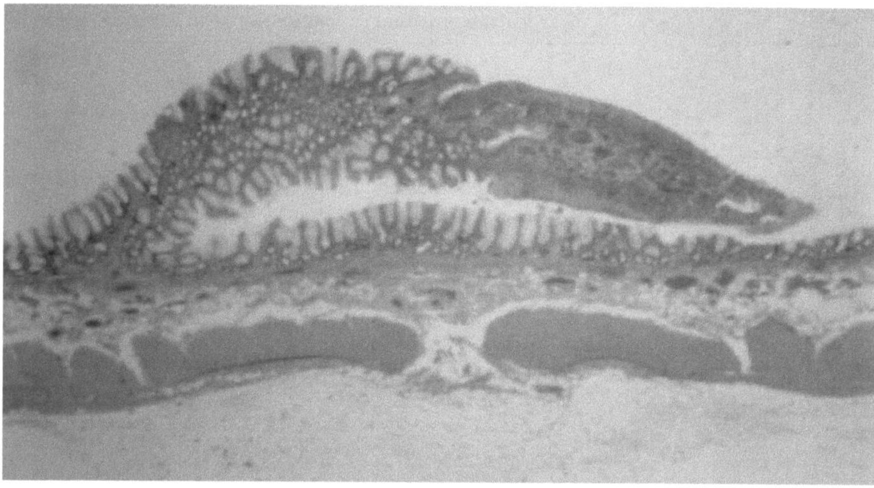

Figure 8 A case of cap polyp. This is a regenerative-type polyp

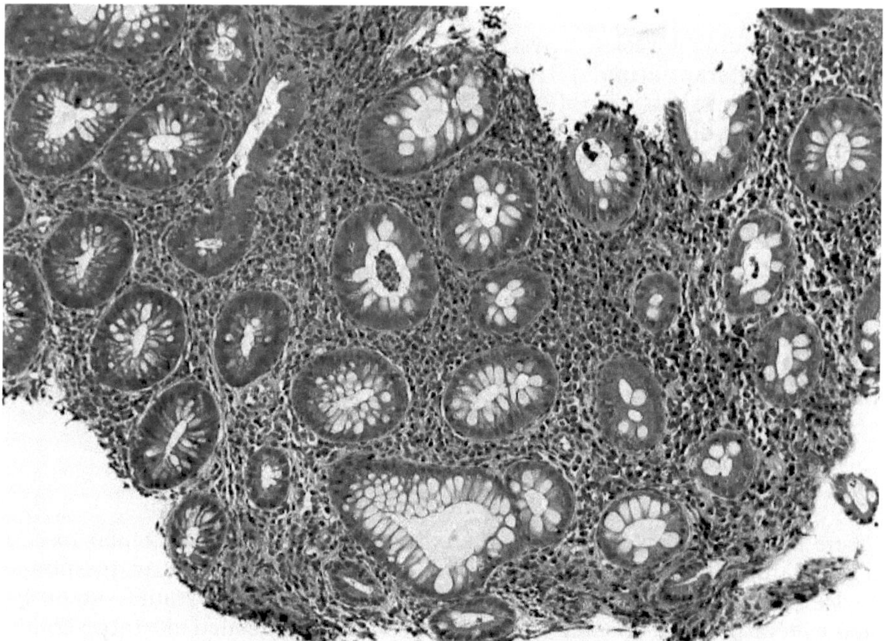

Figure 9 Tear and diamond-shaped crypt similar to solitary ulcer syndrome is seen in a case of mucosal herniation-type diverticular colitis

Table 1 A literature review of 'diverticular colitis 'and its relationship with ulcerative colitis[4]

Year	*Study*	*No. of patients*	*Number UC-like*	*Number with subsequent classical UC*	*Treatment*
1983	Cawthorn et al	3	3	0	Sulph
1984	Sladen and Filipe	5	3	1	Sulph and steroids
1992	Gore et al	34	11	3	Sulph and steroids
1992	Peppercorn	8	8	0	Sulph and steroids
1993	Polit	1	1	0	Sulph and steroids
1995	Hart et al.	14	5	0	Sulph
1996	Van Rosenthal and Andersen	2	2	0	Sulph and antibiotics
1996	Makapugay and Dean	23	23	3	Sulph, antibiotics and steroids
1998	Pereitra	1	1	1	Surgery and medical treatment
2002	Gupta and Shepherd	7	7	0	Surgery
	Total	98	64	8	

Total patient number 98; age range 32–87; sex ratio, M:F = 2:1.
UC, ulcerative colitis; sulph, sulphasalazine, 5-aminosalicylic acid or similar compound.

symptoms within 4 weeks[2,9]. Systemic corticosteroids are rarely required which helps in differentiating it from Crohn's disease, in which steroids and immunosuppressants are often necessary[17]. The duration of inflammatory bowel disease-directed therapy ranges from a month to 4 years[3]. A small proportion of patients with the features of DC will eventually develop classical ulcerative colitis[2]. However, this progression into ulcerative colitis should be considered the exception rather than the rule[2,3,9,16].

Patients with persistent or recurrent symptoms should be considered for sigmoid resection[10]. It has been found that there is a statistically significant increase in the requirement for surgical resection among patients with diverticular disease-associated chronic colitis[3], which led to the assumption that the presence of active chronic colitis of luminal surface mucosa predisposes to the necessity for surgical intervention in diverticular disease[3].

OUTCOME

There is huge debate concerning the correlation between diverticular disease and inflammatory bowel diseases, and there is always a particular question as to whether it is one or two diseases. Although there are a few studies (about 10) in the literature with documented cases of DC with associated ulcerative colitis-like changes, the number of patients who subsequently developed classic ulcerative colitis was eight out of 98 cases[4]. It is very important in suspected cases of DC to have additional biopsies from the rectum and areas more proximal to the affected segment to rule out ulcerative colitis and have a baseline biopsy to study disease progression.

As already mentioned, one of histopathological features of DC might suggest Crohn's disease, such as focal active inflammation, abnormal crypt architecture, and the presence of sarcoid-type granulomas. However, several studies have indicated the patients with DC with such microscopic features more often than not do not progress to the clinical subsequent 'classic' Crohn's disease. The Gledhill and Dixon, and the Burroughs et al. studies both have 17 cases of DC with Crohn's-like features[14,18]. Those have been followed up, and only two cases subsequently developed Crohn's disease.

What is applicable for Crohn's disease is also applicable for ulcerative colitis. Only a few cases of DC have progressed to distal ulcerative colitis.

We believe that there is a single disease, diverticulosis, which may be complicated or influenced by other factors in inducing microscopic changes similar to those often seen in ulcerative colitis and Crohn's disease to give the clinical, endoscopic and histological picture of DC. In some cases, however, two diseases may coexist. Both diverticular disease and inflammatory bowel disease are extremely common, and the presence of one entity would not necessarily ensure protection from another common disease.

MAIN POINTS

1. DC is a rare disease.

2. There is an overlap in symptoms between DC and diverticular disease; however, some cases are subclinical.

3. It is important that clinicians check to rule out inflammatory bowel diseases by performing a biopsy in other parts of the colon, and following up the patients.

4. It is difficult for pathologists to make a definite diagnosis as inflammatory bowel diseases in cases of diverticular diseases. Usually these require a multidisciplinary meeting to sort out such cases. However, there is a strong recommendation for clinicians to follow up these cases.

5. Once established, DC can be divided histologically into three types: ulcerative colitis-like, Crohn's disease-like and mucosal polypoidal types. Whether there is a clinical correlation between the various types is not clear.

References

1. White CL, Hamilton SR, Diamond MP, Cameron JL. Crohn's disease and ulcerative colitis in the same patient. Gut. 1983;24:857–62.
2. Gore S, Shepherd NA, Wilkinson SP. Endoscopic crescentic fold disease of the sigmoid colon: the clinical and histopathological spectrum of a distinctive endoscopic appearance. Int J Colorectal Dis. 1992;7:76–81.
3. Makapugay LM, Dean PJ. Diverticular disease-associated chronic colitis. Am J Surg Pathol. 1996;20:94–102.

4. Ludeman L, Shepherd NA. What is diverticular colitis? Pathology. 2002;34:568–72 (Review).
5. Meyers MA, Alonso DR, Morson B, Bartram C. Pathogenesis of diverticulitis complicating granulomatous colitis. Gastroenterology. 1978;74:24–31.
6. Goldstein NS, Leon-Armin C, Mani A. Crohn's colitis-like changes in sigmoid diverticulitis specimens are usually an idiosyncratic inflammatory response to the diverticulosis rather than Crohn's colitis. Am J Surg Pathol. 2000;24:668–75.
7. Goldstein NS, Ahmad E. Histology of the mucosa in sigmoid colon specimens with diverticular disease: observations for the interpretation of sigmoid colonoscopic biopsy specimens. Am J Clin Pathol. 1997;107:438–44.
8. Ludeman L, Warren BF, Shepherd NA. The pathology of diverticular disease. Best Pract Res Clin Gastroenterol. 2002;16:543–62 (Review).
9. Peppercorn MA. Drug-responsive chronic segmental colitis associated with diverticula: a clinical syndrome in the elderly. Am J Gastroenterol. 1992;87:609–12.
10. Rampton DS. Diverticular colitis: diagnosis and management. Colorectal Dis. 2001;3:149–53.
11. Imperiali G, Meucci G, Alvisi C et al. Segmental colitis associated with diverticula: a prospective study. Am J Gastroenterol. 2000;95:1014–16.
12. Jani N, Finkelstein S, Blumberg D, Regueiro M. Segmental colitis associated with diverticulosis. Dig Dis Sci. 2002;47:1175–81.
13. Shanahan F, Bernstien CM. ANCAs aweigh in colitis. Gastroenterology. 1993;105:946–7.
14. Gledhill A, Dixon MF. Crohn's-like reaction in diverticular disease. Gut. 1998;42:392–5.
15. Kelly JK. Polypoid prolapsing mucosal folds in diverticular disease. Am J Surg Pathol. 1991;15:871.
16. Hart J, Baert F, Hanauer S. Sigmoiditis: a clinical syndrome with a spectrum of pathological features, including a distinctive form of IBD. Mod Pathol. 1995;8:62A.
17. Guslandi M. Segmental colitis: so what? Euro J Gastroenterol Hepatol. 2003;15:11–12.
18. Burroughs SH, Bowrey DJ, Morris-Stiff GJ, Williams GT. Granulomatous inflammation in sigmoid diverticulitis: two diseases or one? Histopathology. 1998;33:349–53.

2
Pathogenesis of diverticular disease: enteric neuropathy

T. WEDEL, M. BÖTTNER and H.-J. KRAMMER

INTRODUCTION

The first description of diverticular disease dates back over more than 300 years, when Littre reported 'saccular outpouchings of the colon' in 1700 (cited in ref. 1). About 100 years later Graser[2] introduced the terms 'false diverticula' and 'peridiverticulits', pointing out that the colonic wall prolapse is confined to a herniation of the mucosal and submucosal layers (pseudodiverticula) and frequently associated with subsequent inflammatory reactions. Nowadays, diverticular disease is still considered as a major century-old problem[3], and ranges among the most common diseases affecting the colon in Western countries.

However, in spite of the clinically and socioeconomically important impact of this condition our understanding of the underlying pathogenesis is still incomplete – most likely because the aetiology cannot be simply reduced to a single pathophysiological mechanism but rather appears to be multifactorial. The most widely accepted and traditionally propagated concepts concerning the pathogenesis of diverticular disease involve ageing, dietary habits, and both structural and functional alterations of the colonic wall.

CLASSICAL PATHOGENETIC CONCEPTS

Ageing

It is evident from epidemiological studies that a higher age clearly favours the development of diverticula[4–6]. Whereas this condition is uncommon under the age of 40, the prevalence increases rapidly from approximately 20% at the age of 50 to around 60% at the age of 70. Although advancing age is obviously associated with diverticular disease, this association may be ostensible, as it is not age *per se*, but the prolonged time-course during which the colonic wall is exposed and therefore more susceptible to other pathogenetic factors (see below).

Diet

Data from both clinical studies and experimental animal models have shown that a low fibre intake correlates positively with the formation of diverticula[6,7]. It has been suggested that a lack of dietary fibre delays colonic transit time[8] and produces smaller stool amounts due to increased water absorption, thereby diminishing the luminal diameter. According to the law of Laplace a smaller radius will result in higher intraluminal pressure and, hence, facilitate the development of diverticula[9]. Although dietary fibre has been proven to be protective against these alterations, there is no clear evidence for a benefit of a high-fibre intake in asymptomatic diverticular disease to prevent the onset of symptoms[10].

More recently, dietary fibre has also been discussed regarding its effects on the colonic bacterial flora and their fermentation products (e.g. short-chain fatty acids)[11]. Thus, in fibre-deficient rats the concentration of short-chain fatty acids was considerably lower, and has been suggested to induce connective tissue alterations of the colonic wall resulting in a higher incidence of diverticula[7,10]. In contrast, other dietary habits, such as smoking and the intake of alcohol or caffeine, are not correlated with an increased risk of symptomatic diverticular disease[12].

Structural alterations of the colonic wall

Beside luminal factors, changes of the colonic wall itself have also been suggested to cause diverticula. The corresponding studies have focused on structural alterations of either the connective tissue or the intestinal musculature. Two major extracellular matrix components, collagen and elastin, have been found to be altered in diverticular disease: smaller, more densely packed collagen fibrils and an excessive crosslinking of collagen molecules with increased rigidity and a subsequent loss of tensile strength[13,14], and an increase of elastic fibres (elastosis) confined to the longitudinal muscle layer with a subsequent thickening of the colonic wall[15]. Indeed, thickening of the muscular layers has been shown to be a typical feature in diverticular disease[16]. However, the increase in muscle tissue could not be attributed either to hypertrophy or to hyperplasia, but appeared to be related to a considerable shortening of the colonic wall due its contractile state ('myochosis').

Functional alterations of the colonic wall

The most accepted pathophysiological common final pathway resulting in mucosal herniation appears to be increased intraluminal pressure. It is thought that excessive segmental contractions transform the colonic wall into concertina- or bladder-like compartments ('bladder colon') causing both a functional obstruction and painful sensations. Evidence for disturbed motility patterns is mainly derived from manometric and myoelectric studies showing that patients with diverticular disease, particularly those with a symptomatic course, are characterized by higher intracolonic pressure and increased motility indices after administration of meals or provocative pharmacological agents such as morphine or prostigmine[17–21]. As most of the early investigations were biased by inconsistant methodological approaches (e.g. patient selection, anatomical site of recording, time period of recording), other studies have focused on those colonic segments truly affected by diverticula[22,23], and have prolonged the recording time[24], revealing that diverticular disease is associated with increased motor activity and high-amplitude propagated contractions.

ENTERIC NEUROPATHY – A NEGLECTED ENTITY IN DIVERTICULAR DISEASE?

Overall, the data obtained from functional studies support a disturbed colonic motility as one of the main pathophysiological mechanisms underlying diverticular disease. Given that the enteric nervous system primarily accounts for the mediation of normal intestinal motility, and has been shown to be affected in a broad spectrum of colonic motility disorders[25,26], it is surprising that studies on intestinal innervation in diverticular disease are rather scarce.

Morphological alterations of the enteric nervous system

The first communication regarding histopathological alterations of the enteric nervous system in diverticular disease originated from Macbeth and Hawthorne[27] in 1965. They described enlarged myenteric ganglia mainly due to an increase in glial cells and ectopic ganglia located within the muscle layers, suggesting that diverticular disease is not defined merely by a muscular dysfunction but also by neural tissue alterations ('acquired neuromuscular derangement'). Ten years later Morson[28] confirmed an increase in neural tissue but attributed the changes to a shortening of the colonic wall frequently observed in diverticular disease.

Stoss and Meier-Ruge[29] have primarily focused on the submucous plexus and described hypertrophied nerve fibre strands and so-called submucous giant ganglia, both features resembling what has been defined by Meier-Ruge as intestinal neuronal dysplasia[30]. It was postulated that a deranged submucous plexus hampers the reflex circuits required for coordinated peristalsis, resulting in disturbed motility patterns and, hence, in the development of diverticula.

Vuong et al.[31] were not able to confirm these structural alterations previously reported in patients with diverticular disease. However, their study was limited to the myenteric plexus and based on either conventional histological or silver impregnation staining techniques, the latter not being suitable to visualize the entire population of enteric neurons.

More recently we investigated the enteric nerve plexus in transmural sections and whole-mount preparations obtained from patients with diverticular disease by means of nerve-specific immunohistochemical techniques (pan-neuronal marker Protein Gene Product 9.5)[32]. With respect to controls, the enteric nervous system of patients with diverticular disease displayed a lesser neuronal content within myenteric ganglia in 25% of cases (oligoneuronal hypoganglionosis) and hypertrophied submucous nerve fibre strands and ganglia in 16% of cases, the latter finding being compatible with the histopathological features of intestinal neuronal dysplasia. The alterations were most impressive in those colonic segments affected by diverticula. In constrast to previous studies, the neuropathological lesions were apparent only in a subgroup of patients with diverticular disease, most likely reflecting the clinical heterogeneity of the patients. Nevertheless, the observed decrease in myenteric nerve cells displayed similarities to other conditions, such as slow-transit constipation or idiopathic megacolon, in which the functional intestinal obstruction could be linked to an oligoneuronal hypoganglionosis of the myenteric plexus[33,34]. Thus, it is likely that in diverticular disease a deranged enteric nervous system may contribute to intestinal motor disturbances, thereby predisposing to the development of diverticula.

Using the same pan-neuronal antibody Simpson and colleagues[35] found an enhanced nerve tissue staining within the circular muscle layer in patients with both acute and chronic diverticulitis, the latter group additionally characterized by increased mucosal nerve fibres. In line with observations in animal models of experimental colitis[36,37], they suggested that, after an initial loss of mucosal nerves, a proliferative nerve remodelling and regenerative hyperinnervation of the musculature may be induced in response to inflammation.

Alterations of neurotransmitters

Besides structural alterations of the enteric nervous system some studies also assessed the expression status of neurotransmitters released by enteric neurons. Milner et al.[38] found an increased level of the neurotransmitter vasoactive intestinal polypeptide in patients with diverticular disease, and speculated that a disturbed neurotransmitter homeostasis is likely to contribute to a disturbed colonic transit.

In a more recent study peridiverticular mucosal biopsies were assessed for expression levels of tachykinins (substance P, neuropeptide K) and galanin in asymptomatic and symptomatic patients with diverticular disease (Simpson et al., abstract presented at the Association of Surgeons of Great Britain and Ireland, Manchester, 2003). Interestingly, tachykinins and galanin were up-regulated in those patients with painful diverticular disease, implying their involvement in the generation of symptoms due to an injury of the enteric nervous system possibly mediated by previous or ongoing inflammatory events. Based on their own findings, and data from experimental colitis and clinical studies in patients with irritable bowel syndrome, Simpson et al.[39] suggested in a recent review that the concept of visceral hypersensitivity (excessive perception of physiological stimuli with increased reflex responses) may also hold true for the origin of symptoms in diverticular disease. They postulated 'that the hypersensitivity originates locally, possibly as a result of nerve damage following acute diverticulits ... providing plausible mechanisms for the generation of gastrointestinal symptoms'.

In-vitro studies

Further evidence for a functionally altered enteric nervous system is given by *in-vitro* studies assessing the contractility of smooth muscle strips in response to nerval stimulation. Performing isometric tension experiments, Tomita et al.[40,41] have shown that, after stimulation of enteric nerves, smooth muscle strips obtained from patients with diverticular disease contract more frequently and are less able to relax in response to vasoactive intestinal polypeptide and NO donors. Moreover, exogenously administered acetylcholine resulted in an increased sensitivity[42] and uncoordinated muscle contraction[43] in patients with diverticular disease. However, in contrast to previous studies, Golder et al.[42] have attributed the hypersensitivity to acetylcholine not to an increased, but decreased, cholinergic innervation with a compensatory up-regulation of muscarinergic (M3) receptors.

Again, similar to the results of Spiller and colleagues[39], Golder et al.[42] emphasized the previously documented[44] overlap in physiological abnormalities between diverticular disease and irritable bowel syndrome, suggesting common pathological effector mechanisms for both diseases. As patients with the latter disorder are more likely to develop diverticula[45] it was stated that 'for these reasons, the idea of a prediverticular disorder, in which bowel-wall motility is high, before development of diverticula, has been widely accepted'[42].

CONCLUSIONS

Although classical pathogenetic concepts rightly suggest that colonic diverticular disease is related to advancing age, dietary habits and connective tissue alterations of the bowel wall, there is an increasing body of evidence for an involvement of the enteric nervous system in this disease. Morphological and functional data could readily demonstrate that enteric nerves are affected in diverticular disease, and may therefore contribute to both the generation of symptoms and disturbed motor functions leading to abnormal peristalsis patterns and, hence, the development of diverticula.

It is probably not yet justified to consider the documented enteric neuropathy as a reason to propose a paradigm change concerning the pathogenesis of diverticular disease. The heterogeneity of this condition (e.g. left versus right diverticulosis, early versus late onset of diverticulosis, asymptomatic versus symptomatic course, abnormal versus unaltered colonic motility patterns) makes it difficult to encircle the aetiology to a single event. However, an appraisal of the enteric nervous system appears to be a promising field for both basic and clinical research to further clarify its involvement in the pathogenesis of diverticular disease. In particular, a more detailed analysis of the nature of intrinsic intestinal innervation disorders underlying this condition will help to identify more targeted therapeutic approaches – both in terms of the prevention of diverticula and the alleviation of symptoms.

References

1. Finney JMT. Diverticulitis and its surgical treatment. Proceedings of the Inter-State Post-Graduate Medical Assembly of North America, 1928;55:57–65.
2. Graser E. Das falsche Darmdivertikel. Münch Med Wochenschr. 1899;22:721–3.
3. Schoetz DJ Jr. Diverticular disease of the colon: a century-old problem. Dis Colon Rectum. 1999;42:703–9.
4. Parks TG. Post-mortem studies on the colon with special reference to diverticular disease. Proc R Soc Med. 1968;61:932–4.
5. Hughes LE. Postmortem survey of diverticular disease of the colon. II. The muscular abnormality of the sigmoid colon. Gut. 1969;10:344–51.
6. Gear JS, Ware A, Fursdon P et al. Symptomless diverticular disease and intake of dietary fibre. Lancet. 1979;1:511–14.
7. Wess L, Eastwood M, Busuttil A, Edwards C, Miller A. An association between maternal diet and colonic diverticulosis in an animal model. Gut. 1996;39:423–7.
8. Burkitt DP, Walker AR, Painter NS. Effect of dietary fibre on stools and the transit-times, and its role in the causation of disease. Lancet. 1972;2:1408–12.
9. Painter NS, Truelove SC, Ardran GM, Tuckey M. Segmentatiion and the localization of intraluminal pressures in the human colon, with special reference to the pathogenesis of colonic diverticula. Gastroenterology. 1965;49:169–77.
10. Wess L, Eastwood MA, Edwards CA, Busuttil A, Miller A. Collagen alteration in an animal model of colonic diverticulosis. Gut. 1996;38:701–6.
11. Bengmark S. Ecological control of the gastrointestinal tract. The role of probiotic flora. Gut. 1998;42:2–7.
12. Aldoori WH, Giovannucci EL, Rimm EB, Wing AL, Trichopoulos DV, Willett WC. A prospective study of alcohol, smoking, caffeine, and the risk of symptomatic diverticular disease in men. Ann Epidemiol. 1995;5:221–8.
13. Wess L, Eastwood MA, Wess TJ, Busuttil A, Miller A. Crosslinking of collagen is increased in colonic diverticulosis. Gut. 1995;37:91–4.
14. Thomson HJ, Busuttil A, Eastwood MA, Smith AN, Elton RA. The submucosa of the human colon. J Ultrastruct Mol Struct Res. 1986;96:22–30.
15. Whiteway J, Morson BC. Elastosis in diverticular disease of the sigmoid colon. Gut. 1985; 26:258–66.
16. Morson BC. The muscle abnormality in diverticular disease of the colon. Proc R Soc Med. 1963;56:798–800.
17. Arfwidsson S, Knock NG, Lehmann L, Winberg T. Pathogenesis of multiple diverticula of the sigmoid colon in diverticular disease. Acta Chir Scand. 1964;63(Suppl. 68).
18. Painter NS, Truelove SC, Rdran GM, Tuckey M. Effect of morphine, prostigmine, pethidine, and probanthine on the human colon in diverticulosis studied by intraluminal pressure recording and cineradiography. Gut. 1965;28:57–63.
19. Parks TG, Connell AM. Motility studies in diverticular disease of the colon. Gut. 1969;10: 534–42.
20. Ritsema GH, Thijn CJ, Smout AJ. [Motility of the sigmoid in irritable bowel syndrome and colonic diverticulosis.] Ned Tijdschr Geneeskd. 1990;134:1398–401.
21. Weinreich J, Andersen D. Intraluminal pressure in the sigmoid colon. II. Patients with sigmoid diverticula and related conditions. Scand J Gastroenterol. 1976;11:581–6.
22. Trotman IF, Misiewicz JJ. Sigmoid motility in diverticular disease and the irritable bowel syndrome. Gut. 1988;29:218–22.
23. Cortesini C, Pantalone D. Usefulness of colonic motility study in identifying patients at risk for complicated diverticular disease. Dis Colon Rectum. 1991;34:339–42.
24. Bassotti G, Battaglia E, Spinozzi F, Pelli MA, Tonini M. Twenty-four hour recordings of colonic motility in patients with diverticular disease: evidence for abnormal motility and propulsive activity. Dis Colon Rectum. 2001;44:1814–20.
25. Goyal RK, Hirano I. The enteric nervous system. N Engl J Med. 1996;334:1106–15.
26. Schemann M, Neunlist M. The human enteric nervous system. Neurogastroenterol Motil. 2004;16(Suppl. 1):55–9.
27. Macbeth WA, Hawthorne JH. Intramural ganglia in diverticular disease of the colon. J Clin Pathol. 1965;18:40–2.

28. Morson BC. Pathology of diverticular disease of the colon. Clin Gastroenterol. 1975;4:37–52.
29. Stoss F, Meier-Ruge W. Diagnosis of neuronal colonic dysplasia in primary chronic constipation and sigmoid diverticulosis endoscopic biopsy and enzyme-histochemical examination. Surg Endosc. 1991;5:146–9.
30. Meier-Ruge W, Gambazzi F, Kaufeler RE, Schmid P, Schmidt CP. The neuropathological diagnosis of neuronal intestinal dysplasia (NID B). Eur J Pediatr Surg. 1994;4:267–73.
31. Vuong NP, Sezeur A, Balaton A, Malafosse M, Camilleri JP. [Myenteric plexuses and colonic diverticulosis: results of a histological study.] Gastroenterol Clin Biol. 1985;9:434–6.
32. Wedel T, Roblick UJ, Schiedeck TH, Bruch HP, Krammer HJ. Ist die Divertikelkrankheit mit intestinalen Innervationsstörungen assoziiert? Viszeralchirurgie. 1999;34:307–11.
33. Wedel T, Roblick UJ, Ott V et al. Oligoneuronal hypoganglionosis in patients with idiopathic slow-transit constipation. Dis Colon Rectum. 2002;45:54–62.
34. Wedel T, Spiegler J, Soellner S et al. Enteric nerves and interstitial cells of Cajal are altered in patients with slow-transit constipation and megacolon. Gastroenterology. 2002;123:1459–67.
35. Simpson J, Haji-Suyoi A, Jenkins D, Schoefield JH, Spiller RC. Quantification of neurological changes in resection specimens with complicated and uncomplicated diverticular disease. Gastroenterology. 2002;122:A314 (abstract).
36. Stead RH. Nerve remodelling during intestinal inflammation. Ann NY Acad Sci. 1992;664:443–55.
37. Sanovic S, Lamb DP, Blennerhassett MG. Damage to the enteric nervous system in experimental colitis. Am J Pathol. 1999;155:1051–7.
38. Milner P, Crowe R, Kamm MA, Lennard-Jones JE, Burnstock G. Vasoactive intestinal polypeptide levels in sigmoid colon in idiopathic constipation and diverticular disease. Gastroenterology. 1990;99:666–75.
39. Simpson J, Scholefield JH, Spiller RC. Origin of symptoms in diverticular disease. Br J Surg. 2003;90:899–908.
40. Tomita R, Munakata K, Aoki N, Tanjoh K, Kurosu Y. A study on the peptidergic nerves (VIP, substance P) in the colon of patients with diverticular disease. Regul Pept. 1993;46:244–6.
41. Tomita R, Fujisaki S, Tanjoh K, Fukuzawa M. Role of nitric oxide in the left-sided colon of patients with diverticular disease. Hepatogastroenterology. 2000;47:692–6.
42. Golder M, Burleigh DE, Belai A et al. Smooth muscle cholinergic denervation hypersensitivity in diverticular disease. Lancet. 2003;361:1945–51.
43. Huizinga JD, Waterfall WE, Stern HS. Abnormal response to cholinergic stimulation in the circular muscle layer of the human colon in diverticular disease. Scand J Gastroenterol. 1999;34:683–8.
44. Otte JJ, Larsen L, Andersen JR. Irritable bowel syndrome and symptomatic diverticular disease – different diseases? Am J Gastroenterol. 1986;81:529–31.
45. Havia T, Manner R. The irritable colon syndrome. A follow-up study with special reference to the development of diverticula. Acta Chir Scand. 1971;137:569–72.

3
Pathogenesis of diverticular disease: altered motility

M. E. KREIS

INTRODUCTION

Diverticular disease has a rising incidence since it occurs mainly in the elderly population and, in general, the average age of the population increases in developed countries[1]. Consequently, this condition becomes more relevant, and has therefore received increasing attention in recent years.

The pathogenesis of diverticula in the human colon and associated diseases such as inflammation and bleeding are mainly unknown. One reason may be that suitable animal models to study the pathophysiology are missing. Most clinicians are familiar with the concept that diverticular disease is associated with increased intraluminal pressures in the sigmoid colon and that removal of the 'high-pressure zone' by sigmoid colectomy usually cures the patient. At first sight it appears to be logical that increased intraluminal pressures may trigger herniations of the intestinal mucosa through the muscle layers of the colon, leading to diverticula (Figure 1). However, the number of studies investigating this aspect of diverticular disease is very limited. The aim of this brief review is to summarize the available evidence as regards alterations in colonic motility associated with diverticular disease, and to discuss its role in the disease progress.

METHODS

The review was based on a literature search from the Medline database from 1966 until May 2005. Only original articles presenting data from colonic manometry studies in patients and volunteers were included. When comparing studies, particular attention was paid to data on the colonic motility index in response to a standard meal and the acetylcholinesterase inhibitor neostigmine, as well as to high-amplitude propagated contractions in the colon.

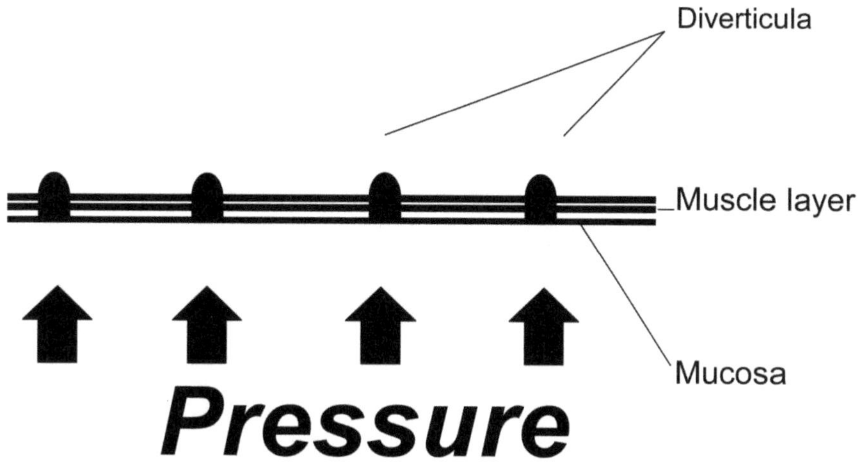

Figure 1 Schematic view to illustrate the theoretical concept of how increased intraluminal pressure may contribute to the formation of diverticula

RESULTS

Colonic motility at baseline, i.e. without a stimulus, was compared between patients with diverticular disease and healthy controls in several studies[2–5] (Table 1). Only Trotman and Misiewicz found a difference in colonic motility index under baseline conditions; however, they did not report the raw data in their investigation[4]. The remaining studies described similar colonic motility indices in patients with diverticular disease and controls[3–5]. One limitation of these reports is that the groups of patients with diverticular disease were not well defined. This is overcome in a more detailed investigation by Cortesini et al.[6] who differentiated four subgroups: controls, patients with asymptomatic diverticular disease (diverticula without symptoms), patients wtih uncomplicated symptomatic diverticular disease (diverticula with left lower quadrant pain) and patients with symptomatic complicated diverticular disease (diverticula and complications such as haemorrhage, diverticulitis, bowel obstruction, or fistulas). Interestingly, under basal conditions, and following a standard meal, only patients with uncomplicated and complicated symptomatic diverticular disease had an increased colonic motility index during manometry in the sigmoid colon, but not patients with asymptomatic diverticula (Figure 2). It appears that increased intraluminal pressures were mainly associated with symptoms secondary to colonic diverticula rather than the diverticula themselves.

Attisha and Smith, as well as Weinreich et al., recorded the colonic motility index following administration of neostigmine in patients with diverticular disease[3,7]. Both studies found that patients with diverticular disease have an increased response to neostigmine compared to controls.

Table 1 Studies comparing the colonic motility index as determined by manometry between controls and patients with diverticular disease

Study	*Controls (n)*	*Diverticular disease (n)*	*p-Value*
Parks and Connell 1969[2]	528 (15)	470 (25)	n.s.
Attisha and Smith 1969[3]	151 (9)	343 (29)	n.s.
Trotman and Misiewicz 1988[4]	Not given (13)	Not given (6)	<0.02
Katschinski et al. 1990[5]	379/224–636 (13)	282/209–394 (15)	n.s.

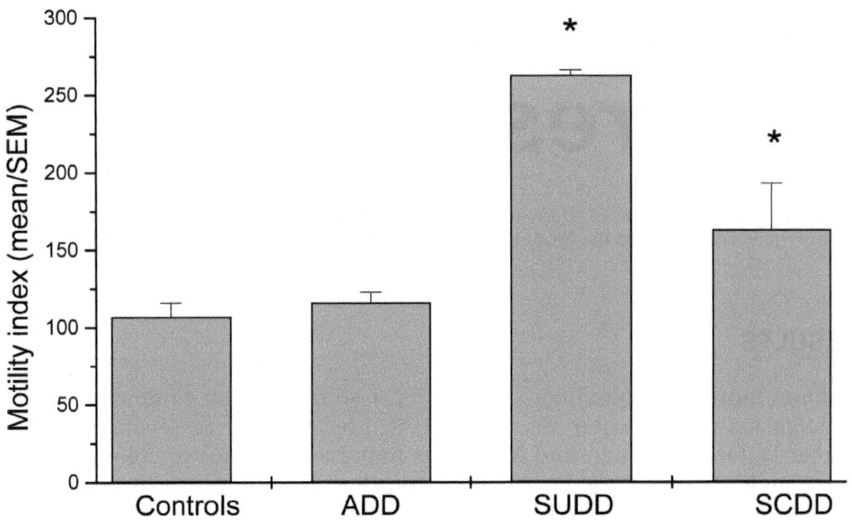

Figure 2 Comparison of the motility index during baseline colonic manometry recordings in specific subgroups of patients with diverticula and controls. Controls: patients without diverticula (n = 30); ADD: patients with asymptomatic diverticula (n = 30); SUDD: patients with symptomatic uncomplicated diverticular disease (n = 30); SCDD: patients with symptomatic complicated diverticular disease (n = 55). *$p < 0.001$ (from ref 6).

In 2001 Bassotti et al. published a comparative investigation of colonic motility in patients with symptomatic uncomplicated diverticular disease and controls[8]. In this study colonic motility was recorded for 24 h, which allowed the authors not only to quantify motor events but also to analyse motility patterns. They found that the characteristic high-amplitude propagated contractions occurred almost twice as often in patients compared to controls. Furthermore, 20 % of this activity was retrogradely propagated in patients with diverticular disease, which was never observed in controls. Another remarkable finding of this intriguing study was that all motility abnormalities were confined to the diseased segment, suggesting that diverticular disease is not necessarily a disorder of the entire colon. In a more recent study Bassotti et al. reported that patients with diverticulosis had prolonged periods of phasic pressure activity compared to controls[9]. Interestingly, periods of phasic pressure activity were associated with crampy abdominal pain.

Apart from simply comparing patients with diverticular disease and controls, other groups went further and explored the question of whether altered colonic motility may be reversed following treatment of diverticular disease. This is the case when myotomy is undertaken in order to reduce the increased pressure in the sigmoid colon when diverticular disease is present[3]. Of course, this investigation is historical, as myotomy is no longer performed to treat diverticular disease, but following sigmoid colectomy colonic pressures are also reduced[10]. In a different study, conservative treatment of diverticular disease was investigated by switching the patients to a high-fibre diet. Here, it was similiarly found that intraluminal pressures were decreased in the sigmoid colon[11].

DISCUSSION

The concept that altered motility is associated with diverticular disease is supported by a panel of studies highlighting different aspects of this condition. First, the prevalence of this disorder increases with age[1]. In parallel, segmental contractile activity in the colon also increases with age[12], which may be related to ageing of colonic smooth muscle[13]. Second, Cortesini and others reported patients with symptomatic diverticular disease as displaying a higher colonic motility index during manometry when compared to patients carrying diverticula without symptoms[6]. Third, the abnormal motility was reduced following surgery[3,10]. These studies and others clearly indicate that diverticular disease involves alterations in colonic motor activity.

It is of note that most studies needed either test stimuli such as neostigmine or a standard meal, or a very detailed analysis of prolonged recordings of motor events in order to delineate differences in colonic motility between patients and controls. This may be explained either by the substantial variation that occurs when colonic motility is recorded, or by the hypothesis that differences between patients and controls are very subtle. Furthermore it appears that alterations in colonic motility are limited to patients with symptomatic diverticula, but do not occur in patients with asymptomatic diverticula. This observation suggests that the motility disorder is not a causative factor for the generation of diverticula but rather a consequence of changes secondary to their presence such as recurrent inflammation. In contrast, the observation that switching the patients' diet to high fibre content reduces intraluminal pressures in the sigmoid colon supports the hypothesis that a low-fibre diet with subsequent high colonic pressures contributes to the generation of diverticula[11].

In conclusion, there is evidence that symptomatic diverticular disease is associated with increased pressure peaks in the colon, prolonged periods of elevated intraluminal pressure and altered patterns of colonic motility. It remains to be determined, however, whether these alterations of colonic motility are causing the later development of colonic diverticula or whether they are rather secondary to structural changes in the colonic wall subsequent to diverticular disease.

SUMMARY

The pathophysiology of diverticular disease is not well understood. Studies investigating alterations in colonic motility associated with diverticular disease were mostly undertaken in patients. Manometry recordings in the sigmoid colon demonstrated that pressures recorded in the lumen are generally higher in patients with diverticula compared to controls, especially following stimuli such as a standard meal or neostigmine. A particular association with increased intraluminal pressures appears to be present in patients who suffer from symptoms and who have complicated forms of diverticular disease. Furthermore, the pattern of colonic motility is altered in a substantial proportion of patients. Surgery and conservative treatment with a high-fibre diet appears to reduce the increased intraluminal pressures in diverticular disease. Whether altered motility causes the development of diverticula, or whether it is merely an epiphenomenon of structural changes in the colon secondary to the disease, remains to be determined.

References

1. Almy TP, Howell DA. Diverticular disease of the colon. N Engl J Med. 1980;302:324–31.
2. Parks TG, Connell AM. Motility studies in diverticular disease of the colon. Gut. 1969;10: 534–42.
3. Attisha RP, Smith AN. Pressure activity of the colon and rectum in diverticular disease before and after sigmoid myotomy. Br J Surg. 1969;56:891–4.
4. Trotman IF, Misiewicz JJ. Sigmoid motility in diverticular disease and the irritable bowel syndrome. Gut. 1988;29:218–22.
5. Katschinski M, Lederer P, Ellermann A, Ganzleben R, Lux G, Arnold R. Myoelectric and manometric patterns of human rectosigmoid colon in irritable bowel syndrome and diverticulosis. Scand J Gastroenterol. 1990;25:761–8.
6. Cortesini C, Pantalone D. Usefulness of colonic motility study in identifying patients at risk for complicated diverticular disease. Dis Colon Rectum. 1991;34:339–42.
7. Weinreich J, Andersen D. Intraluminal pressure in the sigmoid colon. II. Patients with sigmoid diverticula and related conditions. Scand J Gastroenterol. 1976;11:581–6.
8. Bassotti G, Battaglia E, Spinozzi F, Pelli MA, Tonini M. Twenty-four hour recordings of colonic motility in patients with diverticular disease. Dis Colon Rectum. 2001;44:1814–20.
9. Bassotti G, Battaglia E, De Roberto G, Morelli A, Tonini M, Villanacci V. Alterations in colonic motility and relationship to pain in colonic diverticulosis. Clin Gastroenterol Hepatol. 2005;3:248–53.
10. Cortesini C, Bruno L, Pantalone D. Motility effects of anterior resection of the rectum performed for diverticular disease. Ital J Surg Sci. 1989;19:369–73.
11. Hodgson J. Effect of methylcellulose on rectal and colonic pressures in treatment of diverticular disease. Br Med J. 1972;3:729–31.
12. DiLorenzo C, Florres AF, Hyman PE. Age-related changes in colon motility. J Pediatr. 1995;127:593–6.
13. Butt Wg, Wang M, Kaufmann ST. Age-related changes in rat colon mechanics. J Gastrointest Motil. 1993;5:121–8.

4
Pathogenesis of diverticular disease: genetic disposition versus the environment

A. FORBES

INTRODUCTION

Diverticulosis affects more than 50% of those aged over 60 in Western populations. Given that diverticulosis is relatively rare in African and traditional Asian populations it is unsurprising that during much of the latter part of the 20th century the condition was attributed to low-fibre diets, and to the prolonged colonic transit time and increased intraluminal pressure associated with low-volume stools. These factors have been said to be responsible for pulsion diverticula (which are not true diverticula), which emerge through the circular layer of the muscularis propria at points of penetration of the vasa recta that supply the submucosa and mucosa. It is also maintained that the diverticula occur as a result of primary weakness of the colon wall and that abnormalities of collagen may be implicated. Colonic diverticulosis is associated with altered collagen content and the expression of tissue inhibitor of metalloproteinases, which may play a role in remodelling the gut wall in this condition[1].

EPIDEMIOLOGY AND POPULATION CHANGE

As a primitive population at low risk of diverticular disease alters its behaviour to become more like that of the affluent North and West the condition begins to emerge. It coincides with adoption of a Western-type refined diet but also independently with a move from rural to urban living[2]. It is remarkably difficult to perform interventional studies in this area and we are left with a major question in respect of causality.

The Japan to Hawaii migration studies showed a dramatic (1% to 50%) increase in diverticulosis with the more Western environment (and lower fibre intake)[3]. However, much of this increase was in the right-sided disease that is more prevalent in the Japanese remaining in Japan[3]. While this confirms that an environmental element is important, it does not negate the importance of the genetic component. The disease characterization and its significance are addressed in more detail elsewhere in this volume. Suffice it to say that, on available evidence, the genetic component appears to be stronger in right-sided diverticulosis than in left-sided disease.

The remarkable Singapore autopsy study of 1986 remains a benchmark in diverticulosis research[4]. No fewer than 1014 consecutive adult intestines were examined, and diverticulosis was found in 19%. There were more affected women in the under-60-year age group, but most striking was the racial differentiation. Although Singapore covers a very small area, and is in some ways a cohesive community, there are three major population groups with different culture and customs, and of course different genetic backgrounds. Diverticulosis was considerably commoner in men of Chinese origin than those of Indian ($p<0.002$) or Malay ($p<0.01$) origin.

DIVERTICULAR DISEASE AND DIET

If it is accepted that diet is important it is implicit that there must be an underlying mechanism or series of mechanisms. Unfortunately few data exist to assist in their analysis in respect of diverticulosis. In other contexts there are now many observations that the nature of the food eaten influences the colonic luminal content, directly and through its influence on the qualitative and quantitative effects on the colonic microflora. There is also a little evidence to suggest that dietary fibre has an impact on the collagen and elastin content of the colon wall[5].

The fibre content of the diet can easily be shown to affect transit time, and, with a little extrapolation, fibre content can be shown to influence intraluminal pressure in line with the law of Laplace (explored elsewhere in this volume). It is possible that fibre has an influence on protection of the colonic wall from toxic elements, but there are no data specific to this in respect of diverticulosis.

ANIMAL MODELS

Diverticular disease can be induced in a number of animal models and this phenomenon has been most often exploited in the rat. Prolonged feeding of a low-fibre diet will provoke the formation of colonic diverticula, and this is prevented by a high-fibre diet[6]. This is probably in part at least the result of an effect on collagen crosslinking, which occurs to a much lesser extent in animals on a high fibre intake[5]. However, there are many important differences between the pathophysiology of the rat and that of humans; not least among which is the symmetry of the muscle layers in the rat colon which therefore lacks taeniae. The rabbit, which like us has a taenial colon, can be induced to develop diverticular disease but only with some difficulty, and only if the animal is also treated with anticholinesterases[7]. Issues concerning the electrophysiology of the colon will be addressed by others in this volume and will not be considered any further here.

FAMILY STUDIES

It is clear that low-fibre intake cannot be the full explanation for the development of diverticulosis, and family studies have indicated that there is likely to be a genetic component to the risk of developing the condition. However, it must be conceded that the literature is thin indeed. For 'family studies' one should really read 'case reports'. There have been isolated reports describing the condition affecting (for example) multiple siblings (perforating sigmoid diverticulitis in a pair of German monozygotic twins[8]; diverticular disease in three Italian sisters[9]; complicated diverticular disease in two young adult brothers in the UK[10]; severe disease requiring resection before the age of 30 in another pair of monozygotic twins[11]; and in three Nigerian siblings[12]).

The young adult siblings of the Nigerian family[12] are especially interesting as, of course, they reflect a population group in whom the condition is normally rare (if increasingly prevalent). However, the three siblings had spent some years in the more industrialized world and environmental factors are not excluded.

There do not appear to be any formal epidemiological family studies that would permit a more confident interpretation.

Studies of rat families provide an interesting diversion, as newborn rats fed a low-fibre diet developed diverticulosis, but at a lower frequency and to a lesser severity than in those born to mothers themselves on a high-fibre diet[13]. While this suggests perhaps an element of Lamarckian evolution, there is also an intriguing human case report that provides an alternative hypothesis.

Perz-Atayde et al. report a 14-year-old with multiple gastrointestinal diverticula, including those in the colon, together with many other muscle problems (smooth and skeletal)[14]. Rectal biopsy led to the diagnosis of a respiratory chain defect which was traced by molecular genetic techniques to have its origin in severe damage to the mitochondrial DNA to be found in ganglia and muscle cells. Mitochondria are, of course, inherited from the mother.

AGE

Diverticulosis predominantly affects the elderly, and is associated with reduced strength of the colonic wall. The mechanisms underlying this remain somewhat obscure but are beginning to be elucidated. It is frequently found that there are fewer collagen fibres between the muscle layers of the colon wall, but that these collagen fibres are abnormally thickened. More paradoxically there is an increase both in elastin content and in the overall thickness of the muscle layer thickness[15].

It appears that most of the pathological changes seen in diverticular disease reflect consequences of the disease, and perhaps especially the consequences of a prior episode of acute diverticulitis, but there is evidence that certain aspects predate the formation of the diverticula themselves. Both increased elastin content of the taeniae and diffuse thickening of the muscle layer can be shown to come first. Colonic wall weakness is most probably an early element and can often affect many areas of apparently unaffected colon in established cases[15].

CONNECTIVE TISSUE DISEASE AND DIVERTICULOSIS

It should now be no surprise to learn that diverticulosis is associated with a range of primary connective tissue disorders. Several of these conditions have a strong genetic component to their aetiology. Interestingly most of the published reports concentrate on non-colonic diverticula (e.g. duodenal and oesophageal, as well as those of non-gastrointestinal organs). It is unclear whether this is an indication of a strong association with non-colonic diverticula, or merely a reflection of colonic involvement seeming less interesting as it is so common in the general population. There is a potential problem here, as publication bias may mean that such cases fail to cross the threshold for case reporting.

Marfan's syndrome has not recently been linked with diverticulosis in published reports but historical reports make the link clear. The pathogenesis of the underlying condition has now emerged, and it appears that most of the autosomal dominant inheritance is via mutations of the FBN1 gene which codes for fibrillin-1[16]. Fibrillin-1 is present in the wall of the healthy colon, but does not yet appear to have been studied in patients with Marfan's.

The Ehlers–Danlos syndromes form a group of connective tissue disorders responsible for abnormal elasticity of the skin and hypermotility of the joints. The most common mutations implicated are those of the COL5A1 gene[17] which codes for collagen 5, which, again, is present in the wall of the healthy colon, but has not yet been studied in patients with Ehlers–Danlos[18].

RENAL DISEASE

It has been suggested that colonic diverticulosis is particularly associated with the polycystic kidney syndromes. Almost all the good work in this area comes from a single group, however[19,20], and following initially reported prevalences as high as 83% (only 10 patients), they have settled on a background prevalence of diverticulosis between 21%[21] and 47%[22], despite dealing with a young group of patients (mean age at death of only 59 years). The diverticulosis does not seem to contribute directly to the excess mortality in polycystic renal disease.

It does not appear that there is a link with the polycystic gene sites identified on chromosome 4, but it is possible that the polycystic gene on the short arm of chromosome 16 is important, there being at least linkage disequilibrium between the two conditions[19].

The very wide range of quoted prevalence of diverticulosis in polycystic disease, even from within a single centre, probably reflects confounding from the strong association of diverticulosis with end-stage renal failure, which clearly often complicates the polycystic syndrome. The prevalence of diverticulosis is probably somewhat greater than 50% in patients with end-stage renal failure without a polycystic syndrome[22]. The dominant effect is therefore more probably an environmental or disease-related association. The mechanism for this association remains speculative. The possibility that immunosuppression is contributory is not supported by direct data, and the relative rarity of diverticula in Crohn's disease in which there is innate and (often) therapeutic immunosuppression is not supportive of such an hypothesis.

CONCLUSIONS

It is clear that much work has yet to be done on the aetiology and pathogenesis of diverticulosis. At present it would be reasonable to conclude that there is strongly suggestive evidence in favour of joint responsibility of genetic and environmental factors. The limited data which exist suggest that right-sided diverticular disease is proportionately more determined by genetic factors than is the case for left-sided disease. Associations with other conditions in which connective tissue is unequivocally abnormal suggest that primary defects of connective tissue (and possibly of muscle) may prove to be the principal aetiological agent in some (rare) cases.

References

1. Mimura T, Bateman AC, Lee RL et al. Up-regulation of collagen and tissue inhibitors of matrix metalloproteinase in colonic diverticular disease. Dis Colon Rectum. 2004;47:371–8.
2. Segal I, Solomon A, Hunt JA. Emergence of diverticular disease in the urban South African black. Gastroenterology. 1977;72:215–19.
3. Sato E, Ouchi A, Sasano N, Ishidate T. Polyps and diverticulosis of large bowel in autopsy population of Akita prefecture, compared with Miyagi. High risk for colorectal cancer in Japan. Cancer. 1976;37:1316–21.
4. Lee YS. Diverticular disease of the large bowel in Singapore. An autopsy survey. Dis Colon Rectum. 1986;29:330–5.
5. Wess L, Eastwood MA, Edwards CA, Busuttil A, Miller A. Collagen alteration in an animal model of colonic diverticulosis. Gut. 1996;38:701–6.
6. Fisher N, Berry CS, Fearn T, Gregory JA, Hardy J. Cereal dietary fiber consumption and diverticular disease: a lifespan study in rats. Am J Clin Nutr. 1985;42:788–804.
7. Hodgson WJ. An interim report on the production of colonic diverticula in the rabbit. Gut. 1972;13:802–4.
8. Pusch HH, Borger G, Hirth L, Benkmann HG, Goedde HW. Perforating sigmoid diverticulitis in monozygotic twins. Munch Med Wochenschr. 1979;121:947–8.
9. Vigoni A, Marcato M, Lo Monaco GP, Mandelli L, Omodei-Zorini D. Diverticulosis and diverticular disease (reference to a case of diverticular disease observed in 3 sisters). Chir Ital. 1985;37:656–9.
10. Grainger R, Edwards MH. Complicated colonic diverticular disease in two young adult brothers. J R Coll Surg Edinb. 1987;32:255–6.
11. Frieden JH, Morgenstern L. Sigmoid diverticulitis in identical twins. Dig Dis Sci. 1985;30: 182–3.
12. Omojola MF, Mangete E. Diverticula of the colon in three Nigerian siblings. Trop Geog Med. 1988;40:54–7.
13. Wess L, Eastwood M, Bussutil A, Edwards C, Miller A. An association between maternal diet and colonic diverticulosis in an animal model. Gut. 1996;39:423–7.
14. Perez-Atayde AR, Fox V, Teitelbaum JE et al. Mitochondrial neurogastrointestinal encephalomyopathy: diagnosis by rectal biopsy. Am J Surg Pathol. 1998;22:1141–7.
15. Watters DA, Smith AN, Eastwood MA, Anderson KC, Elton RA, Mugerwa JW. Mechanical properties of the colon: comparison of the features of the African and European colon *in vitro*. Gut. 1985;26:384–92.
16. Booms P, Pregla R, Ney A et al. RGD-containing fibrillin-1 fragments upregulate matrix metalloproteinase expression in cell culture: a potential factor in the pathogenesis of the Marfan syndrome. Hum Genet. 2005;116:51–61.
17. Schwarze U, Atkinson M, Hoffman GG, Greenspan DS, Byers PH. Nul alleles of the COL5A1 gene of type V collagen are a cause of the classical forms of Ehlers–Dnalos syndrome (types I and II). Am J Hum Genet. 2000;66:1757–65.
18. Defuentes G, Damiano J, Moulin O, Hervouet M, Zing E, Berets O. Right diverticular colitis revealing an Ehlers–Danlos syndrome. Presse Med. 2004;33:1591–2.

19. Gabow PA. Autosomal dominant polycystic kidney disease – more than a renal disease. Am J Kidney Dis. 1990;16:403–13.
20. Fick GM, Gabow PA. Natural history of autosomal dominant polycystic kidney disease. Annu Rev Med. 1994;45:23–9.
21. Fick GM, Johnson AM, Hammond WS, Gabow PA. Causes of death in autosomal dominant polycystic kidney disease. J Am Soc Nephrol. 1995;5:2048–56.
22. Sharp CK, Zeligman BE, Johnson AM, Duley I, Gabow PA. Evaluation of colonic diverticular disease in autosomal dominant polycystic kidney disease without end-stage renal disease. Am J Kidney Dis. 1999;34:863–8.

Section II
Clinical issues

Chair: M. ANTHUBER and M. LUKAS

5
Diverticular disease – differential diagnosis and prognosis

S. HOLLERBACH

INTRODUCTION

Diverticulosis of the colon is quite frequent in developed countries and prevalence rises with age. Though up to two-thirds of people older than age 80 years are affected by the presence of diverticula, most of them (70%) remain asymptomatic throughout their entire life. Only up to 30% of patients develop symptoms related to the presence of diverticulosis that consist of either uncomplicated diverticulitis, diverticular haemorrhage, or complicated diverticulitis[1–4] including recurrent diverticulitis, fistula formation, or peritonitis and sepsis. The causes of colonic diverticula include alterations in colonic wall resistance, disordered colonic motility, and dietary deficiencies, particularly fibre and bran. While the frequent left-sided colitis appears to be an acquired disease, right-sided diverticular disease is much less common, can occur at younger age, and appears to be more common in Asians[2–4]. The clinical spectrum of the symptomatic cases that account for approximately only 20–30% of individuals that carry diverticula in the colon[1,2,5,6] ranges from non-specific intermittent abdominal pain to potentially life-threatening complications such as perforating diverticulitis, fistulizing disease, or haemorrhage. Hence, diverticular disease has emerged as a major health problem, particularly in developed countries with an extraordinarily ageing population. In the elderly, diverticular disease has already become the most common colonic disorder and causes significant morbidity and mortality[2–4,7–10]. Colonoscopy, abdominal ultrasound, and helical computed tomography (CT) scanning of the abdomen are the most important tools for diagnosis and clinical management of these patients. Here, I particularly review the differential diagnosis and the prognosis of diverticular disease in light of the different degrees of clinical severity of the disease.

DIFFERENTIAL DIAGNOSIS

To review the differential diagnosis of diverticular disease, we first have to look at the spectrum of clinical symptoms (Table 1). In the elderly individual, diverticular disease is one of the most common colonic disorders and causes significant morbidity and mortality[1–6]. The mere presence of diverticula in the colon, however, is only called asymptomatic diverticulosis, which does not automatically warrant being regarded as an illness unless it eventually becomes symptomatic over time. In symptomatic diverticular disease, however, the complaints and clinical symptoms are rather unspecific, suggesting that other common and uncommon colonic diseases have to be ruled out, in particular since most patients who suffer from diverticular disease are older than 55 years. In this age group the most significant colonic disease that has to be ruled out as the most important differential diagnosis (Table 2a and 2b) is colorectal carcinoma (CRC). CRC has an increasing incidence with age and its precursors (colonic adenomatous polyps) are frequently found accidentally during routine prophylactic colonoscopy in asymptomatic individuals. Diverticular disease and CRC also share common risk factors, particulary older age, lack of physical exercise, fat-enriched and low-fibre diets, and the higher incidence of left-sided colonic disease that may be due to motility disturbances and differences in faecal stream physics (Table 3). Hence, all patients above age 45 years with unspecific complaints in the lower abdomen should definitely undergo colonoscopy to rule out coexisting colonic polyps and CRC, as well as other diagnosis such as inflammatory bowel disease (IBD) and ischaemic or drug-induced chronic colitis.

Table 1 Signs and symptoms of diverticular disease of variable severity

Uncomplicated diverticular disease
Non-specific pain (lower left quadrant)
Bloating, constipation
Loose stools
Change in bowel habits
Complicated diverticular disease
Rectal bleeding
Obstruction
Fever, pyrexia
Frank rebound/guarding

In contrast, the most common differential diagnosis of diverticular disease is irritable bowel syndrome (IBS), which presents with clinical symptoms such as non-specific abdominal pain, bloating, and changes in bowel habits. Recurrent local inflammation can produce very short-lived ‘IBS-like’ symptoms, the ‘typical’ IBS symptomatology differs in terms of its chronicity and recurrent periodic pattern. A clear differential diagnosis on clinical terms only, however, is usually not possible. There may be a pathophysiological link between IBS and diverticular disease, since a coexistence of both syndromes is frequently

Table 2a Major differential diagnosis in diverticular disease

Carcinoma of the colon (CRC)
IBS
IBD
NSAID-induced enterocolitis
Pseudomembranous colitis
Other infectious colitides
Appendicitis
Ischaemic colitis

Table 2b Other differential diagnoses in diverticular disease

Women:
Ovarian cysts/abscess
Adnexitis
Urinary tract infections (UTI)
Nephrolithiasis
Groin hernia (incarcerated)

Table 3 Common risk factors in diverticulosis and colon cancer

Age
Obesity, lack of exercise
Low-fibre diet, fat-enhanced diet (red meat)
Alcohol, nicotine
Reduced colonic diameter + reduced wall compliance
Luminal obstruction (stool, polyps)

reported[3,4]. However, to date no biological marker has been consistently identified to establish the close relationship between IBS and diverticular disease. There is certainly room for meticulous research studies to elucidate these important and presently largely uncharted clinical territories in the near future. Other differential diagnoses of chronic lower abdominal symptoms are other forms of chronic colitis such as ischaemic colitis, non-steroidal anti-inflammatory drug (NSAID)-related chronic enteropathy ('diaphragm disease'), and chronic ovarian or tubar disease in women (Table 2a and 2b). Less common differential diagnoses of diverticular disease include left-sided ovarian processes such as bleeding cysts and tubo-ovarian abscess formation in female patients. In addition, conditions such as adnexitis, urinary tract infection, kidney stones and even groin hernias can sometimes be clinically indistiguishable from diverticulitis, especially in obese patients.

If, however, diverticular disease presents with lower gastrointestinal bleeding, the differential diagnosis becomes wider, including other potentially bleeding conditions such as rectal cancer and polyps, haemorrhoidal disease, NSAID-related colonic and ileal ulcers, ischaemic colitis, and angiodysplasia, as summarized in Table 4. To establish a definite cause of bleeding, colonoscopy is certainly the method of choice in most instances, but other modalities

Table 4 Differential diagnosis of lower gastrointestinal bleeding

Carcinoma of the colon
Colonic polyps
IBD
Infectious colitides
Ischaemic colitis
NSAID enteropathy
Angiodysplasia

including enteroscopy, video capsule endoscopy of the small bowel, and extensive radiological work-up (CT scan, angio-CT, angiography) may be necessary to direct the specific treatment options.

PROGNOSIS OF DIVERTICULAR DISEASE

The prognosis of diverticular disease is largely determined by the severity of its clinical symptoms at initial presentation (Figure 1). In approximately 70% of individuals with diverticula of the colon no symptoms occur during their lifespan. These asymptomatic individuals mostly remain asymptomatic throughout life, and have an excellent prognosis of not becoming an affected patient. Symptomatic patients, however, account for approximately the other subset that includes approximately 30% of individuals with diverticulosis. Their individual prognosis is largely determined by the clinical severity of the disease[1–10]. While a single attack of uncomplicated diverticulitis usually resolves very quickly with conservative treatment only, recurrent disease requires surgery in up to 30–40% of patients affected and the rate of complications, as well as its mortality, can double. Fortunately, only 25–30% of symptomatic patients develop a 'virulent' course of their disease that may lead to the formation of genitourinary fistulas, bowel obstruction, life-threatening haemorrhage, or bowel perforation with peritonitis.

The individual risk factors that affect the rate of symptomatic versus asymptomatic diverticulosis are largely unknown. However, age, obesity, diabetes, and immunosuppression are probably special risk factors that may also affect the severity of diverticulitis in selected patients. In addition, the literature suggests that certain 'high-risk' groups exist that may have a different prognosis[9–16]. The first group consists of patients who present at an age of onset younger than 40 years, who account for 2–5% of cases with diverticulitis. The affected individuals are usually obese males, and they tend to experience a more virulent disease than others, since up to 66–88% of these patients require urgent surgery during their initial attack. In addition, they appear to have a high risk of recurrence of inflammation or complications such as fistulizing disease, bleeding, and obstruction. Obesity can be an important risk factor in these affected young people, as well as their dietary habits. For these reasons, and because of the low operative risk of an elective procedure in an otherwise healthy young patient, surgical resection should be generally considered after

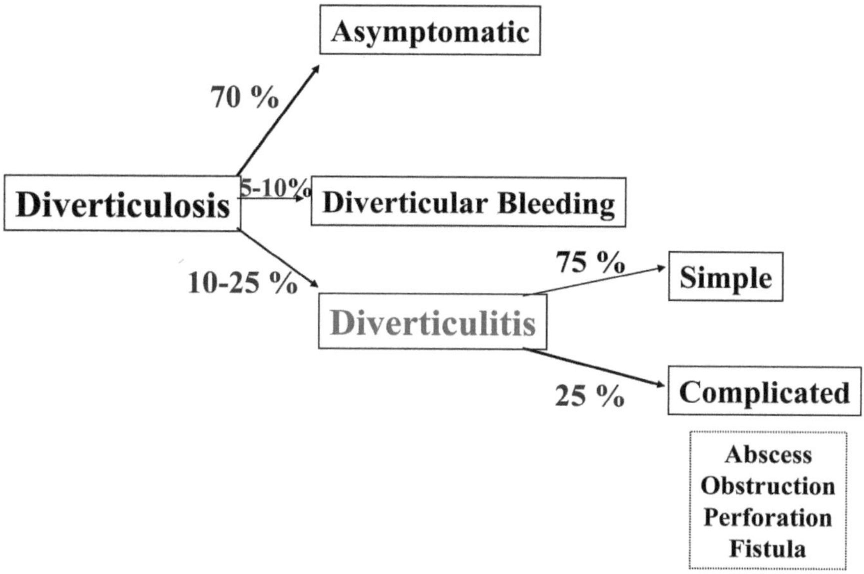

Figure 1 Prognosis of diverticular disease

one well-documented episode of diverticulitis, even if not complicated by confounding factors. However, more recent studies have challenged these preliminary assertions that orginate mainly from the surgical literature. Probably these studies focused on highly selected patients, thus containing a selection bias, suggesting that the results cannot be generalized to all affected patients of younger age. There is a clear need for prospective controlled data in this setting, until clinical guidelines can be established.

Diverticular disease is definitely more virulent in immunocompromised patients, since the disease appears to occur more 'silently' and subtly in this group than in immunocompetent individuals. The morbidity and mortality from diverticulitis appear to be much higher in this subset of patients[15,16]. Such patients can represent a diagnostic challenge, and they are less likely to benefit from conservative medical treatment alone. The key symptoms, such as left lower quadrant pain and fever, may not be present at all, and the only complaint can be fever of unknown origin, which in turn should always provoke a meticulous clinical search for obscure signs of 'silent' diverticulitis in such patients. In addition, they appear to have a higher rate of free abdominal perforation, need for surgery, and postoperative mortality, than immunocompetent individuals. Hence, some authorities advocate elective resection even after one episode of acute diverticulitis in immunocompromised patients, but evidence-based data are largely lacking. There is certainly room, and also a need, for prospective clinical trials in this setting.

SUMMARY AND CONCLUSIONS

Diverticular disease of the colon is clinically indistinguishable from other common and uncommon colonic diseases. Since the majority of patients with symptomatic diverticular disease presents at an age older than 55 years, presence of colon cancer has to be ruled out immediately. Other important colonic diseases that may have the same symptoms include IBS, IBD, drug-induced chronic enterocolitis (NSAID-related) and ischaemic colitis, that can only be reliably assessed by applying modern videoendoscopy with biopsies. In severe cases with abdominal guarding or peritonitis, all other causes of an 'acute abdomen' have to be taken into account, such as acute pancreatitis, gut perforation, perforating ulcer and gallstone disease, and diseases of the genitourinary system. By using modern diagnostic equipment this differential diagnosis can be obtained very quickly in the majority of cases.

The prognosis of symptomatic diverticular disease depends largely on the severity of the disease at the initial attacks, and on the presence or absence of complicating factors. Simple bouts of mild diverticulitis usually respond quickly to medical treatment and have an excellent prognosis, while recurrent or complicated attacks of acute diverticulitis require surgery quite frequently. The surgical mortality (and thereby the prognosis) is largely determined in this subset of patients by factors such as old age, concomitant disease, lack of correct diagnosis, and prolonged time to treatment. Hence, patients with a low risk of elective surgery should undergo an operation after recurrent attacks. The risk of complications is greatest in the presence of comorbidity and in immunocompromised patients. In the latter group special attention is necessary to avoid missing this diagnosis, since the typical clinical symptoms are frequently obscure or missing, while the course of the disease is usually complicated and may lead to a fatal outcome if not detected in time.

References

1. Rose BD. Spectrum and prognosis of diverticulosis and diverticular disease. UpToDate Med. 1997;14:252–7.
2. Stollmann NH, Raskin JB. Diagnosis and management of diverticular disease of the colon in adults: ad hoc practice parameters committee of of the American College of Gastroenterology. Am J Gastroenterol. 1999;94:3110–21.
3. Young-Fadok TM. Course and prognosis of uncomplicated and complicated diverticular disease. Colon Rect Surg. 2001;3:420–4.
4. Dunn G. Diverticulosis and diverticulitis – recent developments. Medscape. 2004 (Internet database: www.medscape.com); 22:35–9.
5. Painter NS, Burkitt DP. Diverticular disease of the colon: a deficiency disease of Western civilization. Br Med J. 1971;2:450–4.
6. Painter NS, Burkitt DP. Diverticular disease of the colon, a 20th century problem. Clin Gastroenterol. 1975;4:3–21.
7. Parks TG. Natural history of diverticular disease of the colon. Clin Gastroenterol. 1975;4: 53–69.
8. Konvolinka CW. Acute diverticulitis under age forty. Am J Surg. 1994;167:562–5.
9. Acosta JA, Grebenc ML, Doberneck RC, McCarthy JD, Fry DE. Colonic diverticular disease in patients 40 years old or younger. Am Surg. 1992;58:605–7.

10. Freischlag J, Bennion RS, Thompson JB Jr. Complications of diverticular disease of the colon in young people. Dis Colon Rectum. 1986;29:639–43.
11. Schauer PR, Ramos R, Ghiatas AA, Sirinek KR. Virulent diverticular disease in young obese men. Am J Surg. 1992;164:443–6.
12. Wong WD, Wexner SD, Lowry A. Practice parameters for the treatment of sigmoid diverticulitis: supporting documentation. Dis Colon Rectum. 2000;43:290–7.
13. Reisman Y, Ziv Y, Kravovic D, Negri M, Wolloch Y, Hallevy A. Diverticulitis: the effect of age and location on the course of disease. Int J Colorectal Dis. 1999;14:250–4.
14. Spivak H, Weinrauch S, Harvey JC, Surick B, Ferstenberg H, Friedmann I. Acute colonic diverticulitis in the young. Dis Colon Rectum. 1997;40:570–4.
15. Perkins JD, Shield CF, Chang FC, Farha GJ. Acute diverticulitis: comparison of treatment in immunocompromised and non-immunocompromised patients. Am J Surg. 1984;148: 745–8.
16. Tyau ES, Prystowski JB, Joehl RJ, Nahrwold DL. Acute diverticulitis: a complicated problem in the immunocompromised patient. Arch Surg. 1991;126:855–8.
17. Zuccaro G. Management of the adult patient with acute lower gastrointestinal bleeding. Am J Gastroenterol. 1998;93:1202–8.

Section III
Diagnosis I

Chair: H. KOOP and H. ZIRNGIBL

6
Diagnosis of diverticular disease in primary care

R. H. JONES

INTRODUCTION

Although diverticular disease is a common condition, for an individual general practitioner it is a surprisingly infrequent diagnosis. A careful review of the literature reveals little primary research in community and general-practice settings on diverticular disease, so that reliable information about the population prevalence of diverticular disease, its incidence and natural course in primary care and the characteristic symptoms at presentation is generally lacking.

In this chapter I will begin by describing the pattern of presentation of abdominal complaints in primary care, and go on to discuss some issues concerning patients' reasons for consultation, the task of primary care physicians in the consultation and relate these to the presentation of lower abdominal pain. I will then describe the differential diagnoses of lower abdominal pain in primary care, explore approaches to making an accurate diagnosis of diverticular disease and, finally, identify a number of topics for further research in this field.

GASTROINTESTINAL PROBLEMS IN PRIMARY CARE

General practitioners in Europe, irrespective of the patient registration system, are likely to see between 120 and 200 patients each week, with numbers being lower and consultation times correspondingly longer in Scandinavian countries and, often, the reverse in southern Europe[1]. About 10% of these patients will consult with either new or on-going gastrointestinal problems, and this proportion of workload is reflected in the fact that, in the UK at least, gastrointestinal problems account for approximately 10% of hospital appointments and admissions[2]. A general practitioner will, therefore, see approximately 12–20 patients, of all ages, each week, with acute and chronic gastrointestinal problems.

Consultation analyses in the UK, such as the Royal College of General Practitioners Morbidity Survey in General Practice[3], indicate that about half of gastrointestinal (GI) problems presented to general practitioners are for upper gastrointestinal symptoms and the other half for lower GI symptoms. The lower GI symptoms include abdominal pain, changes in bowel habit (diarrhoea, constipation and alternation between the two), rectal bleeding, the development of hernias, the discovery of a mass and other symptoms which may eventually turn out to be related to genitourinary and pelvic abnormalities, including pelvic pain and suprapubic pain. A number of these patients present to general practitioners with minor perineal and perianal conditions, such as haemorrhoids and pruritus ani.

This wide range of symptoms is reflected in a broad spectrum of differential diagnoses underlying them. These range from the relatively trivial – food poisoning, travellers' diarrhoea and medication side-effects, the peri-anal and perineal problems mentioned above, and transient, non-specific episodes of constipation and diarrhoea – through more troublesome disorders such as irritable bowel syndrome (IBS) and diverticular disease to more severe conditions such as inflammatory bowel disease (IBD), ischaemic colitis and malignant disease. Other extra-gastrointestinal causes of abdominal pain also need to be borne in mind, and include urinary tract infection, uro-gynaecological problems and, rarely, more exotic causes of abdominal pain such as diabetes, haemoglobinopathies (sickle cell crisis) and porphyria.

Table 1 Differential diagnosis of lower abdominal pain in primary care

Food poisoning/travellers' diarrhoea/medication
Irritable bowel syndrome
Pelvic disorders
Inflammatory bowel disease
Diverticulosis/diverticulitis
Vascular causes, e.g. ischaemic colitis
Malignant disease
Urinary tract infection
Haemoglobinopathies, diabetes, etc.

Patients are likely to present to general practitioners with lower abdominal pain either because it is acute and severe, often amounting a medical or surgical emergency, or because it is more chronic, persistent and troublesome. Clearly the diagnostic approach is quite different in the case of the acute abdomen, which will not be discussed further, although of course, in this condition and in the case of GI haemorrhage, the complications of diverticular disease and diverticulitis form an important part of the differential diagnosis.

Before discussing how general practitioners evaluate patients with chronic abdominal pain, it is worth considering how patients make the decision to consult a physician and how primary care physicians approach the consultation.

THE SYMPTOM ICEBERG

This concept of the symptom iceberg (Figure 1) was originally developed by David Hannay[4], a British general practitioner, and has been applied to a number of conditions, particularly the symptoms of gastro-oesophageal reflux disease by Castell and Johnston in the United States[5]. The concept is important, because the symptom iceberg model provides a framework in which to think about the relationships between health, symptoms and illness and, more importantly, between self-care, primary care and secondary and tertiary care. In the figure the dotted line ('the water line') indicates the transition zone that a person crosses to become a patient. Below the water line symptoms are experienced but tolerated or dealt with without recourse to medical attention, or are absent altogether, in both healthy and presymptomatic individuals. Above the water line the first point of contact with medicine for most patients is primary care (general practice and family medicine), with referral to secondary and tertiary care for more complex and intractable problems. It is worth adding that the patient population on which much medical education is based occupies the tiny areas at the apex of the iceberg; medical students are exposed to a highly selected, patient population.

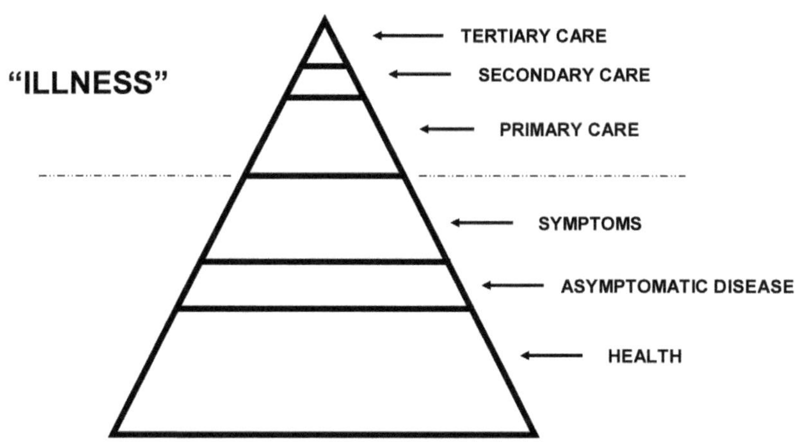

Figure 1 The symptom iceberg

The decision to become a patient is a complex one, and does not depend entirely on symptom severity and the impact of symptoms on work and social activities, but also involves complex decisions about balancing the benefits and costs of declaring one's medical problem and exposing oneself to medical scrutiny, and is also linked to understandings about the likely significance of symptoms – this can work in both directions, so that patients may have inappropriate fears of cancer or heart disease, for example, in gastro-oesophageal reflux disease, or may recognize the potential seriousness of symptoms and, becoming afraid, avoid consultation altogether[6,7].

THE PRIMARY CARE CONSULTATION

The patient emerges from the symptom iceberg and brings to the consultation ideas, concerns and expectations (ICE, as shown in Figure 2). It is essential that the physician explores the patient's ideas of what he/she thinks is happening, and what clues and fears such patients have about their symptoms, their concerns about their symptoms and what sort of problem they may represent and, crucially, the expectations patients have of the medical encounter. The encounter itself consists of a number of partly compartmentalized tasks, which may be addressed sequentially or in varying order, but should always include attention to the acute problem, an appreciation of the background medical history and the presence of chronic problems, an awareness of the opportunities for disease prevention and health promotion and a consideration of the patients' health-care-seeking behaviour; for example, exploring the extent to which patients are taking responsibility for their own illness and are using services appropriately. This model of the primary care consultation was elaborated by Nigel Stott and Robert Harvard Davies in Wales over 20 years ago, and remains a useful framework for consultation analysis[8].

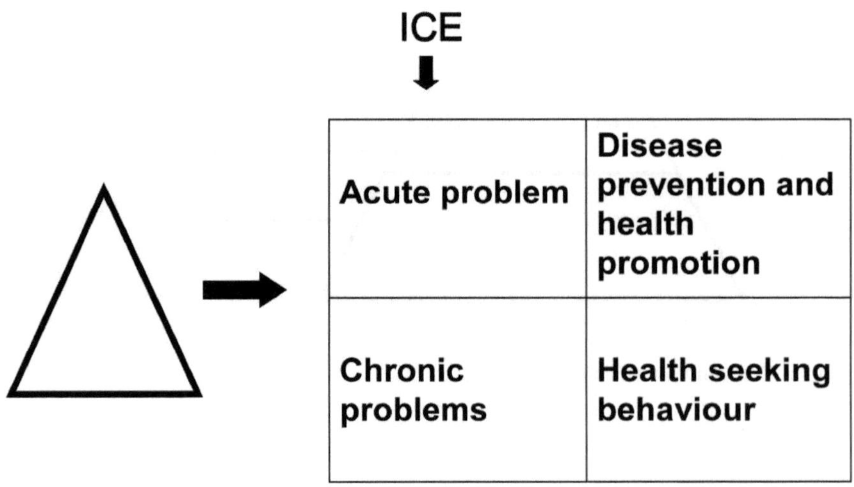

Figure 2 The primary care consultation

Patients may, of course, have obtained a good deal of information about their symptoms before consulting, adding to the lay health beliefs and understandings that are already held. However, it is difficult for patients to obtain useful advice about diverticular disease through internet searches. A Google search on 'diverticulitis' reveals 633 000 results, and over 3 million citations are revealed when 'abdominal pain' is used as the search term. Interestingly, a number of primary care-oriented algorithmic diagnostic websites are unhelpful when it comes to diverticular disease. In the UK, NHS Direct on-line[9] would not have been particularly helpful in making a diagnosis of diverticulitis (although it probably would have ensured that someone with an acute abdominal problem was seen as an emergency at a hospital), and other websites such as familydoctor.org[10], wrongdiagnosis.com[11] (perhaps unsurprisingly), and the American Institute for Preventive Medicine[12] were not particularly helpful in guiding patients towards a diagnosis of diverticular disease, although wrongdiagnosis.com was a helpful site for patients who had already received a diagnosis of diverticular disease.

DIAGNOSTIC DECISION MAKING IN PRIMARY CARE

Marshall Marinker has characterized the roles of generalists and specialists in a helpful way: 'The role of the generalist is to marginalise danger, while that of the specialist is to marginalise uncertainty'[13]. In other words a general practitioner needs to assess a patient, using background knowledge, medical history and clinical examination, to decide whether or not the problem amounts to a condition which requires urgent treatment or investigation, or whether the symptoms amount to considerably less than this and can be dealt with at more leisure, if necessary using time as a therapeutic tool. The specialist, on the other hand, to whom the generalist will have made a referral for an expert opinion, is under pressure to make an accurate, specific diagnosis, and will do his or her utmost to come to a firm diagnostic conclusion either at the first encounter or after further investigation.

Hand-in-hand with this diagnostic approach goes the use of hypothetico-deductive reasoning and pattern recognition in primary care (Table 2), rather than the inductive reasoning approach, based on history, examination and investigations taught to medical students in hospital medicine[14–16]. In reality of course, experts in both hospital and community practice use hypothetico-deductive reasoning and pattern recognition, and also apply general and personal heuristics – often questions or tests thought to have high negative predictive value – to rule in or rule out conditions of concern[17]. A simple example is asking a patient complaining of chest pain whether or not it is related to exertion, as a preliminary screen for likely ischaemic heart disease.

DIAGNOSIS OF DIVERTICULAR DISEASE IN PRIMARY CARE

The key issue for the primary care physician is, essentially, to decide whether a positive diagnosis of diverticular disease can be made in the same way as is

Table 2 Diagnostic decision making in primary care

–	The role of the generalist is to marginalize danger, while that of the specialist is to marginalize uncertainty
–	Hypothetico-deductive reasoning and pattern recognition rather than inductive reasoning are used
–	General and personal heuristic question/tests with high negative predictive value are valuable
–	Clinical epidemiology combined with longitudinal/social familiarity with patient underpins decision making
–	Time is used as a diagnostic tool

generally possible in irritable bowel syndrome (IBS). Although neither the Manning criteria[18] nor the Rome I[19] and Rome II criteria[20] for IBS are based on a mathematical calculation of the sensitivity and specificity or predictive values, of individual symptoms or groups of clinical features, they appear to have acceptable diagnostic precision when correctly applied. It is of interest that most general practitioners are unfamiliar with these criteria yet are still capable of making a positive, symptomatic diagnosis of IBS.

The next question for primary care physicians is whether diverticulosis (without inflammation or complications) can be diagnosed positively in primary care or whether it will always be an incidental finding in someone having contrast radiography or lower bowel endoscopy. The nature of the continuum between diverticulosis and diverticulitis in primary care is poorly understood.

In patients with recurrent abdominal pain suggestive of subacute episodes of diverticulitis, how helpful is abdominal and rectal examination in confirming a diagnosis? What is the role of investigations in these patients? Are there particular alarm symptoms or red flags for referral, short of patients presenting with an acute abdomen.

The approach to diagnosis of chronic abdominal pain in primary care should begin with a careful history, in which the mode and timing of onset is carefully characterized. The pattern of pain, any symptoms associated with pain or pain relief and any other exacerbating or relieving factors all need to be carefully recorded. In taking the history the physician must be guided by the likely differential diagnosis in younger patients (IBS, IBD) and older patients (diverticular disease/diverticulitis, colorectal cancer, vascular disease). It may, however, be very difficult to differentiate some patients with abdominal pain due to diverticular disease from others with the alternating form of IBS and it is unlikely that physical examination, except in acute cases, will add diagnostic precision to the distinction between organic and functional diagnoses.

It is probably reasonable to undertake simple screening investigations such as a full blood count, erythrocyte sedimentation rate (ESR) and C-reactive protein (CRP); the use of investigations in diverticular disease and diverticulitis is discussed elsewhere in this volume, although their diagnostic value in primary care has not been tested.

CONCLUSIONS

For primary care physicians the challenge of making a positive diagnosis of diverticulosis, associated with non-acute episodes of diverticulitis, seems similar to the situation that pertained with IBS 10–20 years ago. This was the time of the emergence of the Manning criteria, which have been superseded by the Rome criteria, and it is perhaps time for similar attention to be paid to patients with diverticular disease. Diverticulosis is less readily considered in the differential diagnosis of lower abdominal pain, although information on the pattern of management in primary care in different parts of the world is lacking.

There is a need for epidemiological research in primary care populations to establish, among other things, the incidence and prevalence of diverticular disease and diverticulitis in these populations, the natural history of the condition, the predictors and correlates of good and bad outcomes in diverticular disease, the utility of alarm symptoms and the links between diverticular disease and symptoms compatible with a clinical diagnosis of IBS.

References

1. Deveugele M, Derese A, van den Brink-Muinen A et al. Consultation length in general practice: cross-sectional study in six European countries. Br Med J. 2002;325:472.
2. Jones R, Murfin D. Gastrointestinal problems in the community and in general practice. In: Jones R, Murfin D, editors. Gastrointestinal Problems in General Practice. Oxford: Oxford University Press, 1993:1–14.
3. Morbidity Statistics for General Practice 1991–92. Royal College of General Practitioners. London: RCGP, 1995.
4. Hannay DR. The Symptom Iceberg. London: Routledge and Kegan Paul, 1979.
5. Castell DO, Johnston BT. Gastroesophageal reflux disease. Current strategies for patient management. Arch Fam Med. 1996;5:221–7.
6. Lydeard S, Jones R. Factors affecting the decision to consult with dyspepsia: comparison of consulters and non-consulters. J Roy Coll Gen Pract. 1989;39:495–8.
7. Crosland A, Jones R. Rectal bleeding: prevalence and consultation behaviour. Br Med J. 1995;311:486–8.
8. Stott NC, Davis RH. The exceptional potential in each primary care consultation. J Roy Coll Gen Pract. 1979;29:201–5.
9. www.nhsdirect.nhs.uk
10. www.familydoctor.org
11. www.wrongdiagnosis.com
12. www.healthylife.com
13. Marinker M. General Practice and the Social Market. London: Social Market Foundation, 1989.
14. Fraser RC, editor. Clinical Method: A General Practice Approach. Oxford: Butterworth–Heinemann, 1999.
15. Baerheim A. The diagnostic process in general practice: has it a two-phase structure? Fam Pract. 2001;18:243–5.
16. Dowie J. Elstein A. Professional Judgement. A Reader in Clinical Decision Making. Cambridge: Cambridge University Press, 1988.
17. Tversky A, Kahnemann D. Judgement under uncertainty: heuristics and biases. Science. 1974;185:1124–31.
18. Talley NJ, Phillips SF, Melton LJ et al. Diagnostic value of the Manning criteria in irritable bowel syndrome. Gut. 1990;31:77–81.
19. Drossman DA, Richter JE, Talley NJ et al. The Functional Gastrointestinal Disorders: Diagnosis, Pathophysiology and Treatment, 1st edition. McLean, VA: Degnon Associates, 1994.

20. Drossman DA, Corazziari E, Talley NJ et al. Rome II. The Functional Gastrointestinal Disorders: Diagnosis, Pathophysiology and Treatment: A Multinational Consensus, 2nd edition. McLean, VA: Degnon Associates, 2000.

7
Laboratory tests – what do they tell us?

C. GASCHE and S. VERMEIRE

INTRODUCTION

The goal of this chapter is to highlight the question of whether laboratory tests may answer relevant clinical questions in patients with uncomplicated diverticular disease, diverticulitis, or complicated diverticulitis. Our task will be first to identify such questions, search for available laboratory tests, and finally separate the 'good from the ugly'.

WHAT RELEVANT QUESTIONS CAN BE RAISED WITHIN THE DIVERSITY OF CLINICAL SITUATIONS IN DIVERTICULAR DISEASE?

The perfect marker would reflect disease extent and the severity of inflammation, it would be independent of therapy unless inflammation decreases, and would be easy to assess and cheap.

Disease extent

As one of the very basic questions, we would like to ask whether diverticula are present at all and, if so, where they are located and how far they extend. To some of our readers this question may sound absurd, since there are obviously no suitable tests available. However, in other disease states (such as inflammatory bowel disease) similar tests have been developed (antineutrophil cytoplasmic antibodies (ANCA) correlate with colonic involvement of IBD, anti-*Saccharomyces cerevisiae* (ASCA) with small bowel involvement; other antibodies such as anti-flagellin or OmpC correlate with tissue penetration or fistulization in Crohn's disease[1]). Even if we do not have a clue how this will be achieved in the future, the question is relevant and appropriate.

Inflammatory disease complication

The second set of questions relates to disease activity and severity. In patients with non-specific bowel symptoms, doctors would like to know whether diverticular disease is uncomplicated, or whether diverticulitis has developed. Furthermore, the severity of diverticulitis, possible penetration/fistulization, or perforation are relevant in patients with acute abdominal pain. This question is much more likely to be answered with current available laboratory tests. The potential candidates are leucocyte counts, blood sedimentation rate, and C-reactive protein. A *Medline Search* on these variables in conjunction with diverticulitis (any term AND diverticulitis; Table 1) revealed an unexpected result: out of 11 original studies that could be identified, the terms leucocyte(s) or leucocytosis were used exclusively to describe study populations rather than to explore the meaning in relation to diverticular disease. This piece of evidence illustrates that clinical trials (imaging or interventional studies) with diverticulitis commonly used elevated leucocyte counts for defining the actual study population. The flipside of the coin, however, reveals an absence of evidence-based studies on the relevance of commonly used laboratory parameters in diverticular inflammation.

Table 1 A Medline search on 'diverticulitis AND common markers of inflammation'

Inflammation marker	*Original*	*Case reports*	*Reviews*	*Non-related*	*Total*
Leukocyte(s)	10	7	9	35	62
CRP	3#	1	–	1	5
ESR or BSR	–	–	1	2	3

#Including two studies already scored in the 'Leukocyte(s)' search.

WHITE BLOOD CELL COUNTS

Increased leucocyte counts are a diagnostic hallmark of diverticulitis. This increase is mainly caused by polymorponuclear cells (neutrophils) rather than lymphocytes. Typical levels in uncomplicated diverticulitis are seen up to 15 000 cells/ml. The mechanism of leucocytosis is partially understood and involves GM-CSF and G-CSF production at the site of inflammation. GM-CSF and G-CSF are important growth factors that stimulate the proliferation and differentiation within the myeloid linage of the bone marrow and cause the circulating leucocyte counts to increase. Other cytokines such as interferons may counteract this mechanism. Normal levels vary between individuals and are influenced by drugs such as corticosteroids (increase) and certain antibiotics or immunomodulators (decrease), which makes this test less sensitive and less specific.

BLOOD SEDIMENTATION RATE

Historically, the separation of blood into fluid and corpuscular elements was first recognized in the eighteenth century. Edmund Biernacki (1866–1912) described in 1897 that the sedimentation rate is increased in sick patients. About 20 years later the method was used as a pregnancy test by Robin Fahraeus (1888–1968) and in 1921 for predicting the prognosis of tuberculosis (Alf Westergren, 1891–1968). It is Alf Westergren's method that is still being used more than 80 years later. The historic development of this test, however, points to the low specificity of the blood sedimentation rate. In our point of view its routine use in diverticulitis is less valuable than leucocyte counts or C-reactive protein levels.

C-REACTIVE PROTEIN

The discovery of C-reactive protein (CRP) followed BSR by less than 10 years. Tillet and Francis from the Rockefeller Institute published a paper in 1930[2] on sera of patients with pneumonia that precipitated with a soluble extract (C-polysaccharide) of *Streptococcus pneumoniae*. This extract was called fraction C, which finally gave the name to C-reactive protein. After resolution of the pneumonia no further precipitation was observed when serum was mixed with fraction C. In patients with a fatal outcome, however, the precipitation reaction remained positive. In the following decades researchers gradually learned that CRP is only one representative of a group of proteins that are regulated during inflammation or systemic stress factors, the so-called acute-phase proteins (Figure 1). These proteins can be divided into positive or negative acute-phase proteins by their ability to increase or reduce expression in response to infection, inflammation, neoplasia, tissue necrosis, or trauma (Table 2). The value of CRP for activity or severity analyses in any infection or inflammatory disease lies in a short half-life (19 h). The only determinant for plasma CRP levels is the *de-novo* synthesis in the liver. An inappropriate CRP response is therefore expected only in chronic liver disease. CRP is not altered by medication unless the underlying disease changes (improves or deteriorates). This is specifically true for diverticulitis, when inflammation is caused by transmural infection with *Escherichia coli* or other commensal gut flora.

Together with the typical clinical presentation of lower left quadrant pain, elevation of these routine laboratory tests is considered to reflect inflammation of diverticula in diverticulitis (Table 3). No studies exist showing that normal levels of these tests preclude diverticulitis. It is likely that microscopic forms of diverticular inflammation do not produce the necessary amount of cytokines that are needed to drive an acute-phase response in the liver or leucocyte generation in the bone marrow. When elevated, these markers correlate with findings of ^{111}indium-labelled leucocyte- and cross-sectional imaging studies. Their significance and superiority in evaluating diverticular inflammation has not been proven.

On the other hand, complications involving bacterial translocation to the peritoneal cavity (perforation or penetration) are associated with a further

DIverticulitis

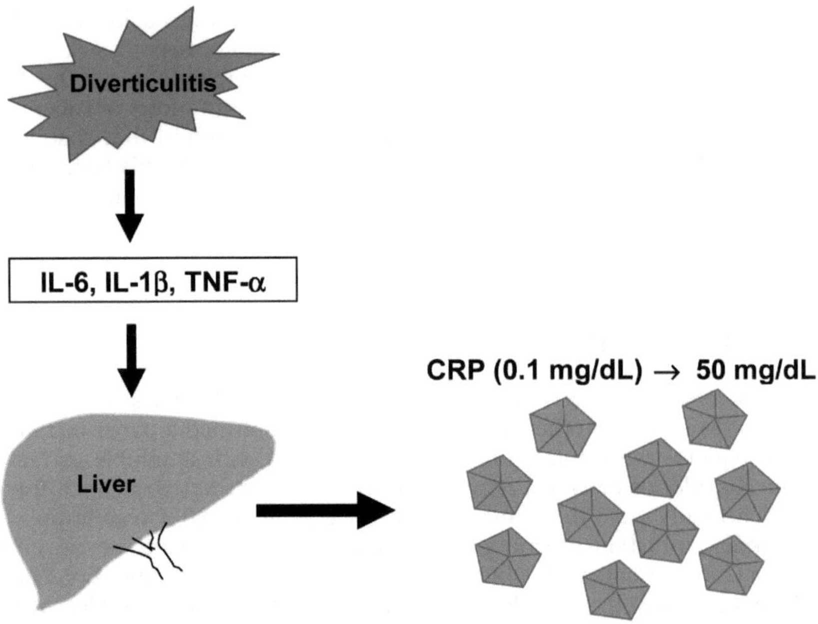

Figure 1 Mechanism of C-reactive protein increase in diverticulitis. As soon as the inflammatory reaction at the site of diverticular inflammation reaches a certain level, it is thought that various immune cells (macrophages, dendritic cells, lymphocytes) produce a variety of soluble cytokines (including IL-β, IL-6 or TNF-α) that may circulate in the blood stream and activate certain receptors and signalling pathways in the liver. Part of this acute-phase reaction is the up-regulation of C-reactive protein synthesis that can be detected within a few hours after the primary stimuli

significant rise in acute-phase response and leucocytes. The reason for this is incompletely understood, but may involve the spread from localized inflammation to a larger area (peritoneal cavity), increased blood flow, specifics of the peritoneal immune response[3], or further translocation of bacteria to the liver or associated sepsis. CRP levels above 20 mg/dl, or leucocyte counts above 20 000 cells/ul, are indicative of peritoneal involvement.

NOVEL LEUCOCYTE-RELATED MARKERS

Faecal calprotectin or lactoferrin have been tested in various forms of inflammatory bowel disease such as Crohn's disease or ulcerative colitis[4]. These ELISA tests measure the concentration of specific leucocyte-related proteins in the stool. Elevated results correlate with the degree of intestinal

Table 2 Acute-phase proteins

	Positive *acute-phase reactants (↑)*	**Negative** *acute-phase reactants (↓)*
Proteinase inhibitors	α_1-**antitrypsin** α_1-antihymotrypsin α_2-macroglobulin	Inter α-antitrypsin
Coagulation/fibrinolysis proteins	**Antithrombin** **Fibrinogen** Prothrombin Factor VIII Plasminogen	
Complement proteins	C1s, C2, B, C3, C4, C5	Properdin
Transport proteins	C1INH Haptoglobin Haemopexin Ceruloplasmin	**Transferrin**
Miscellaneous proteins	**C-reactive protein** Serum amyloid A protein Fibrinonectin α_1-**acid glycoprotein** Gc globulin	**Albumin** Transthyretin High-density lipoprotein Low-density lipoprotein

Table 3 Changes in routine blood tests in diverticulitis

	Change in diverticulitis	*Change in peritonitis*
Leucocytes	↑	↑↑↑
C-reactive protein	↑	↑↑↑
Blood sedimentation rate	↑	↑↑
Haemoglobin	(↓)	(↓)

A drop in haemoglobin is either due to diverticular bleeding (fast drop) or anemia of chronic disease (slow drop)

inflammation and reflect the number of polymorphonuclear cells lost into the faeces through mucosal ulceration or epithelial transmigration. Calprotectin is very stable even at room temperature; lactoferrin is not. They correlate with ^{111}indium-labelled leucocytes; however, their significance and superiority in evaluating diverticular inflammation has not been shown[5,6].

RECURRENCE OF INFLAMMATORY COMPLICATIONS AFTER MEDICAL/SURGICAL THERAPY

A last question that we would like to address deals with recurrence of diverticular disease after surgical resection[7] or diverticulitis after medical therapy. As indicated above, studies on the biological significance of any test in diverticular disease are missing. From the available data it is difficult to draw a definitive conclusion. We have to admit that diverticulitis has never been adequately investigated *per se*, but rather served as 'non-specific inflammatory control' for experimental studies in IBD or colorectal cancer. It is time to spotlight this entity that is commonly associated with morbidity but also mortality.

In conclusion, CRP is the most ideal marker at this moment. There is a great need for studies in diverticular disease assessing its sensitivity to detect complications such as diverticulitis. The best use of CRP at this moment is in the follow-up after start of therapy and in assessing occurrence of complications such as abscess formation.

References

1. Mow WS, Vasiliauskas EA, Lin YC et al. Association of antibody responses to microbial antigens and complications of small bowel Crohn's disease. Gastroenterology. 2004;126: 414–24.
2. Tillet WS, Francis T. Serological reactions in pneumonia with a non-protein somatic fraction of the *Pneumococcus*. J Exp Med. 1930;52:561–71.
3. Russ MA, Reith HB. The severity of infection induces a shift in the type 1/type 2 T-helper cell balance in patients with or without peritonitis. Surg Infect (Larchmt). 2003;4:247–54.
4. Tibble JA, Sigthorsson G, Bridger S, Fagerhol MK, Bjarnason I. Surrogate markers of intestinal inflammation are predictive of relapse in patients with inflammatory bowel disease. Gastroenterology. 2000;119:15–22.
5. Roseth AG, Schmidt PN, Fagerhol MK. Correlation between faecal excretion of indium-111-labelled granulocytes and calprotectin, a granulocyte marker protein, in patients with inflammatory bowel disease. Scand J Gastroenterol. 1999;34:50–4.
6. Saitoh O, Kojima K, Kayazawa M et al. Comparison of tests for fecal lactoferrin and fecal occult blood for colorectal diseases: a prospective pilot study. Intern Med. 2000;39:778–82.
7. Thaler K, Baig MK, Berho M et al. Determinants of recurrence after sigmoid resection for uncomplicated diverticulitis. Dis Colon Rectum. 2003;46:385–8.

8
Lower gastrointestinal bleeding – search for sources

J. SCHÖLMERICH

INTRODUCTION

Lower gastrointestinal (GI) bleeding is defined as acute or chronic blood loss from a source distally to the ligament of Treitz; 10–20% of all GI bleedings belong to this category. The incidence is 25–27/100 000 per year, and there is a strong age dependency. The incidence increases 200-fold from the age of 30 until the age of 90. This is mainly due to bleeding from diverticula and angiodysplasia. Lower bleedings have a less severe course as compared to upper GI bleedings. Mortality is between 2% and 4%, and 80–85% of bleedings stop spontaneously[1]. Among the more severe bleedings diverticular bleedings comprise only one-sixth, while among all bleedings they comprise one-third.

On the contrary, severe haemorrhage can arise in 3–5% of patients with diverticulosis[2,3]. Considering the natural history of diverticular disease 25% of patients have symptoms; of those again 25% have haemorrhages, and of those one-third are massive (Figure 1)[4].

Non-steroidal anti-inflammatory drugs (NSAID) have been implicated in diverticular bleeding pathophysiology. In a large prospective series of patients with lower GI bleeding (50% diverticula) a bleeding risk similar to that in duodenal ulcers has been reported[4,5]. In the Health Professional Follow-Up Study regular NSAID use was associated with an increased risk of diverticular bleeding[6].

CLINICAL FEATURES

Diverticular bleeding usually starts abruptly and without pain. Patients may have mild lower abdominal cramps, followed by passage of voluminous red or dark blood or clots.

In a recent series with 219 patients with lower GI bleeding 41.6% were from diverticula; of those 11% had previous diverticular bleeding; 6.6% needed emergency surgery and hospital mortality was 2.2%. In the survivors after conservative treatment relapse occurred in 9% after 1 year, in 19% after 3 and

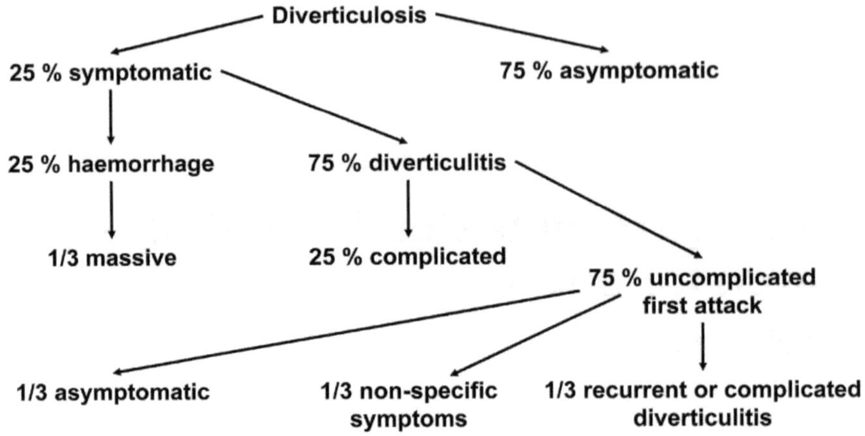

Figure 1 Natural history of diverticulosis and diverticular disease

in 25% after 4 years[7]. In 2005 data on a series of 215 patients with known diverticulosis and severe bleeding have been presented; 13.5% had definitive diverticular haemorrhage, 32% presumed diverticular haemorrhage and 54% incidental diverticulosis[8].

DIAGNOSIS

Upper GI endoscopy is warranted in patients with lower GI bleeding, since 15% of patients with haematochezia will have an upper GI tract cause. Flexible sigmoidoscopy may be used initially to rule out an obvious rectosigmoid lesion, and can be done unprepared. Large series of patients with colonoscopy have been presented, and it was found that 7–10% of patients had significant proximal findings when sigmoidoscopy was normal[9]. Early colonoscopy was associated with short hospitalization in lower GI bleeding as well as with a diverticular source[10].

Emergency colonoscopy in 1561 patients revealed the correct diagnosis in 68% when 13 studies were analysed together[11]. There is no major difference between prepared and unprepared emergency colonoscopy (Table 1); however, earlier series from the 1970s could not demonstrate a difference in mortality as a result of emergency colonoscopy use[12].

With angiography bleeding with an intensity of 0.5–1 ml/min can be detected. An analysis of 14 studies with 764 patients revealed a correct diagnosis in 47% and a complication rate of 9.3% (Table 2)[11]. A comparison between colonoscopy and angiography demonstrated the superiority of the former, although patient numbers were small[13] (Table 3).

Table 1 Diagnosis of lower GI bleeding – emergency colonoscopy[11]

Studies (n)	*Patients (n)*	*Correct diagnosis (n/%)*	*Incomplete examination (n/%)*	*Therapy (n/%)*	*Complications (n/%)*
13	1561	1064/68	36/2	189/12	12/1.3

PREPARATION?

	Correct diagnosis (%)	*Complications (%)*
Prepared	62 (6 studies, 779 patients)	0
Unprepared	76 (3 studies, 461 patients)	1.3

Table 2 Diagnostic investigation in lower GI bleeding – angiography: bleeding up to 0.5–1 ml/min will be detected

Studies (n)	*Patients (n)*	*Correct diagnosis (n/%)*
14	764	359/47

Complication rate 9.3%

Possibility of interventional therapy

	Haemostasis (%)	*Relapse of bleeding (%)*
Embolization	70	0
Vasopressin	71	25

Table 3 Colonoscopy versus angiography in lower GI bleeding[13]

Definitive diagnosis	*Angiography positive*	*Colonoscopy positive*
Angioma	1/5	4/5
Diverticulitis	1/4	3/4
Small intestine lesion	0/3	2/3
Polyp/carcinoma	0/2	2/2
Rectal lesion	0/2	2/2
Endometriosis	0/1	1/1
Total	2/17	14/17

Table 4 Diagnostic investigation in lower GI bleeding – scintigraphy[11]: bleeding up to 0.1 ml/min will be detected

Two methods:		^{99m}Tc colloidal sulphur ^{99m}Tc labelled RBC	
Studies (n)	*Patients (n)*	*Positive scintigram (n/%)*	*Correct diagnosis (n/%)*
16	1418	635/45	269/78*

*95–100% <2 Std, 57–67% >2 Std.

→ if necessary provocation test with heparin??

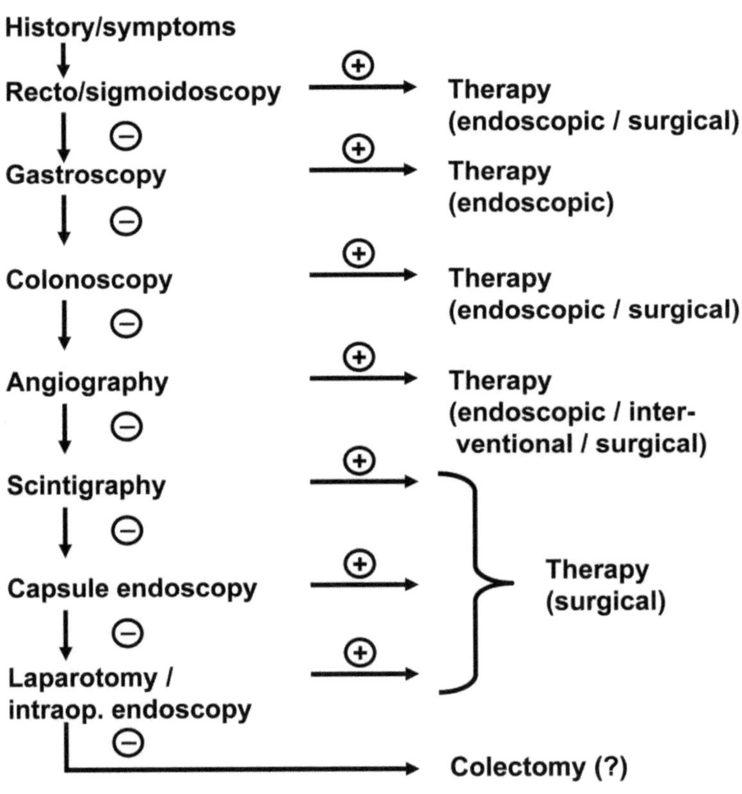

Figure 2 Approach to lower gastrointestinal bleeding

Another alternative is scintigraphy, which has a high sensitivity as compared to angiography regarding the detection of bleeding (cut-off 0.1 ml/min) although it is less good in finding its source[14]. An analysis of 16 studies on 1418 patients revealed a positive scintigram in 45% and a correct diagnosis among those in 78%[11] (Table 4). It may be a useful screening tests prior to angiography[15], but a study did not prove this suggestion[16].

Video capsule endoscopy can be used in patients in whom the upper GI tract and the colon have been eliminated as possible sources. Studies defining its role are still under way – in most centres it is used in order to complete the search for sources in lower GI bleeding[17]. The role of double-balloon endoscopy is currently being tested, while push enteroscopy is less popular and not very effective. Figure 2 gives a possible algorithm for the diagnostic approach to lower GI bleeding.

In summary the available data suggest that diverticular bleeding is a frequent source of lower GI bleeding, and mostly of lesser severity. Emergency endoscopy is most popular and probably useful; it can also be used as treatment. The relapse rate is rather high and elective surgery may be indicated at least after the second bleeding when the diagnosis can be ascertained.

References

1. Messmann HJ, Schölmerich J. Lower intestinal bleeding disorders. In: Classen M, Tytgat GNJ, Lightdale C, editors. Gastrointestinal Endoscopy. Textbook and Atlas. Stuttgart: Thieme Verlag, 2002:598–612.
2. Reinus JF, Brandt LJ. Vascular ectasias and diverticulosis: common causes of lower intestinal bleeding. Gastroenterol Clin N Am. 1994;23:1–20.
3. Zuckerman GR, Prakash C. Acute lower intestinal bleeding: part II – etiology, therapy, and outcomes. Gastrointest Endosc. 1999;49:228–38.
4. Stollman N, Raskin JB. Diverticular disease of the colon. Lancet. 2004;363:631–9.
5. Wilcox CM, Alexander LN, Cotsonis GA, Clark WS. Nonsteroidal anti-inflammatory drugs are associated with both upper and lower gastrointestinal bleeding. Dig Dis Sci. 1997; 42:990–7.
6. Aldoori WH, Giovannucci EL, Rimm EB, Wing AL, Willett WC. Use of acetaminophen and nonsteroidal anti-inflammatory drugs: a prospective study and the risk of symptomatic diverticular disease in men. Arch Fam Med. 1998;7:255–60.
7. Longstreth GF. Epidemiology and outcome of patients hospitalized with acute lower gastrointestinal hemorrhage: a population-based study. Am J Gastroenterol. 1997;92:419–24.
8. Jensen DM, Kovacs TO, Yuan JL, Jensen ME. Inpatient ulcer hemorrhage compared to outpatient hemorrhage: an analysis of prospective cure trials for risk factors, rebleeding, and outcomes. Gastroenterology. 2005;128(Suppl. 2):W1570
9. Mulcahy HE. Yield of colonoscopy in patients with nonacute rectal bleeding: a multicenter database study of 1766 patients. Am J Gastroenterol. 2002;97:328–33
10. Strate L, Syngal S. Early colonoscopy and hospital length of stay in acute lower intestinal bleeding: a nationwide study. Gastrointest Endosc. 2005;61:84 (Abstract).
11. Zuckerman GR, Prakash C. Acute lower intestinal bleeding, part I: clinical presentation and diagnosis. Gastrointest Endosc. 1998;48:477–98.
12. Jensen DM, Machiacado GA, Jutabha R, Kovacs TO. Urgent colonoscopy for the diagnosis and treatment of severe diverticular hemorrhage. N Engl J Med. 2000;342:78–82.
13. Jensen DM, Machicado GA. Diagnosis and treatment of severe hematochezia: the role of urgent colonoscopy after purge. Gastroenterology. 1988;95:1569–74.
14. Hunter JM, Pezim ME. Limited value of technetium 99m-labeled red cell scintigraphy in localization of lower gastrointestinal bleeding. Am J Surg. 1990;159:504–6.

15. Gundermann R, Leef J, Ong K, Reba R, Metz C. Scintigraphic screening prior to visceral arteriography in acute lower gastrointestinal bleeding. J Nucl Med. 1998;39:1081–3.
16. Pennoyer WP, Vignati PV Cohen JL. Mesenteric angiography for lower gastrointestinal hemorrhage: are there predictors for a positive study? Dis Colon Rectum. 1997;40:1014–18.
17. Gölder SK, Schreyer AG, Endlicher E et al. Comparison of capsule endoscopy and magnetic resonance (MR)-enteroclysis in suspected small bowel disease. Int J Colorectal Dis. (In press).

Section IV
Diagnosis II

Chair: C. FOLWACZNY and P. LAYER

9
Intestinal comorbidity: diverticular disease and chronic inflammatory bowel disease

H.-J. KRAMMER, F. SCHLIEGER and T. WEDEL

INTRODUCTION

Sigmoid diverticular disease is common in developed countries and it affects up to half the population (35–60%) over the age of 60 years[1]. Inflammatory bowel disease (IBD) has a second peak of incidence in the elderly[2].

At this second peak Crohn's disease (CD) is more common than ulcerative colitis (UC), and the rectosigmoid is the most common site of active colonic disease[3–6]. It is therefore not surprising that diverticular disease and IBD often coexist; however, Crohn's disease (CD) and diverticulosis coexist more often than would be expected by chance, particularly in elderly women[6–9].

DIVERTICULAR COLITIS

There is increasing recognition of a particular form of IBD that affects the luminal mucosa in the sigmoid colon with diverticular diease[10–14]. Various terms have been given to the condition including: diverticular colitis, segmental colitis, or crescentic colitis. The first of these is the most preferable.

Diverticular colitis is endoscopically characterized by mucosal haemorrhage, disappearance of the vascular reticulum, focal erythema, erosions and ulcers[12].

Histopathological changes vary from non-specific inflammation[11,15] through intense active inflammation with crypt abscesses, and pronounced chronic inflammation, closely mimicking active chronic UC[11–15].

Little is known about the clinical features and natural history of segmental colitis associated with diverticula. Therefore Imperiali et al.[15] performed a large prospective study to evaluate the incidence, clinical presentation and outcome of diverticular colitis. In 5457 colonoscopies 14 patients were found with a segmental colitis associated with diverticula. Haematochezia was the main clinical feature (93%) (Figure 1). The rectum was spared in all cases. Blood chemistry was generally normal and the stool microbiology was negative

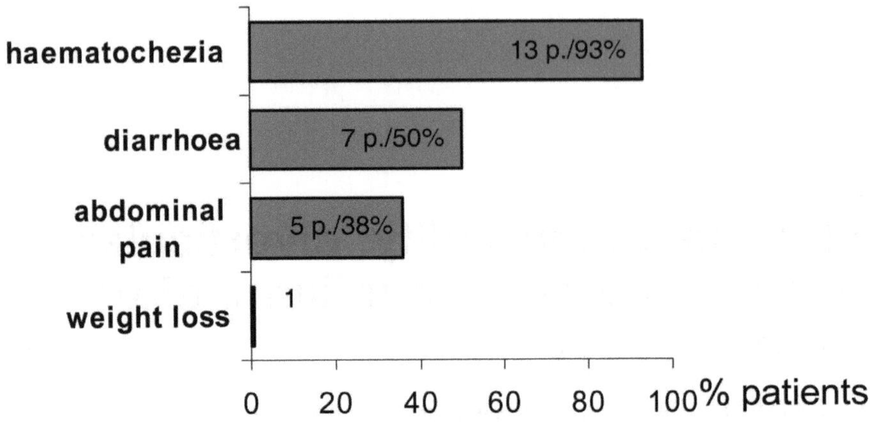

Figure 1 Diverticular colitis: indication for colonoscopy (n = 14)[15]

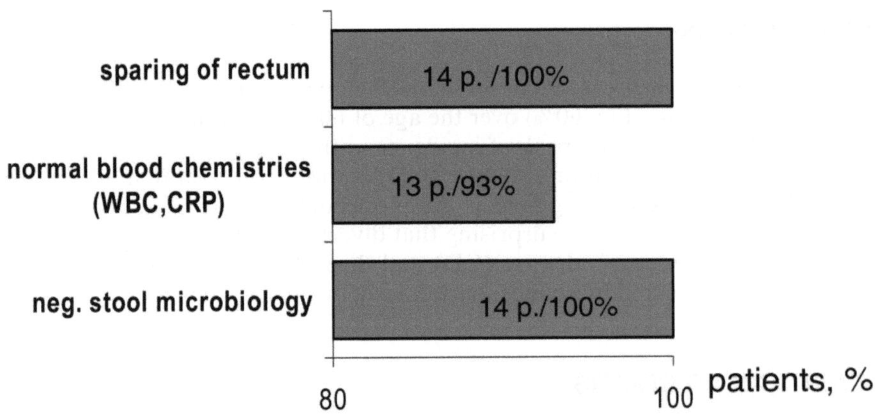

Figure 2 Diverticular colitis: findings[15]

(Figure 2). There was no relation to gender, age, or smoking habits. Diverticular disease has a good clinical outcome and response to treatment similar to that given for IBD. All patients (n = 14) were in clinical and endoscopical remission after 6 weeks treatment with oral and topical 5-ASA.

In conclusion, it is increasingly realized that luminal mucosal inflammation may occur in diverticular disease although, given the frequency of diverticulosis, this form of inflammation seems to be comparatively unusual[11–13]. Diverticular colitis has been associated with various pathogenetic mechanisms, i.e. relative ischaemia of the sigmoid colon, increased exposure to intraluminal antigens and toxins, and changes in bacterial flora related to stasis[11].

DIVERTICULOSIS AND ULCERATIVE COLITIS

While diverticular colitis may closely resemble UC pathologically, in most cases a rectal biopsy specimen is normal and there is no other preceding or subsquent evidence of IBD outside the sigmoid colon[11–14,16,17]. However, there are few cases presenting a diverticular colitis in the sigmoid, with pathological features identical to UC but with endoscopically and histologically normal rectal mucosa, that have subsequently developed classic distal UC with characteristic rectal involvement (Table 1)[11–14]. These patients have responded well to treatment similar to that used in IBD[11–13].

Table 1 Literature review of diverticular colitis and its relationship with UC[19]

Reference	*No. of patients*	*No. with diverticular colitis*	*No. with subsequent classical UC*
Cawthorn et al. 1983[17]	3	3	0
Sladen and Filipe 1984[16]	5	3	1
Gore et al. 1992[11]	34	11	3
Peppercorn 1992[12]	8	8	0
Polit 1993[20]	1	1	0
Hart et al. 1995[14]	14	5	0
Van Rosendaal and Andersen 1996[21]	2	2	0
Makapugay and Dean 1996[13]	23	23	3
Pereira 1998[22]	1	1	1
Gupta and Shepherd 2002	7	7	0
Total	98	64	8

It is possible that these cases of apparent IBD in older patients represent a distinct form of chronic UC, which seems to start in the sigmoid colon affected by diverticular disease and progress to more classic UC.

DIVERTICULOSIS AND CROHN'S DISEASE

In more than 50% of elderly patients with CD there is a concomitant diverticular disease[18]. In the older patient, CD is more likely to affect the distal colon and anorectum than the proximal colon and small bowel[5,6]. The literature would suggest that CD may preferentially involve the colon affected by diverticular disease[7,9]. CD of sigmoid colon may also induce diverticulitis in patients with diverticular disease[8].

The coexistence of CD and diverticular disease seems to carry a worse prognosis, with a more complicated clinical course than either disease by itself. However, it is important to realize that complicated diverticular disease itself may induce pathological changes that are virtually indistinguishable from classical CD affecting the sigmoid colon (Table 2).

Table 2 Diverticular disease and putative mimicry of Crohn's disease (Ludemann et al. 2002)

Reference	*No. of patients*	*Pathology*
Gelb and Finkelstein 1974[23]	1	A, B, C
McCue et al. 1989[9]	4	A, B, C
Naori et al. 1992[24]	3	A, B, C
Gledhill and Dixon 1998[25]	9	A, B, D
Burroughs et al. 1998[26]	8	A, B, C
Goldstein et al. 2000[27]	29	A, B, C, D, E

A, epithelioid granuloma; B, mucosal inflammation; C, aphthous ulcer; D, transmural inflammation; E, fissuring ulceration.

Table 3 Coexistent sigmoid CD-like changes and diverticulitis without prior or concurrent CD in other regions of the bowel[27]

Reference	*No. of patients*	*No. (%) of patients free of post-operative CD*	*Follow-up period (months)*
McCue et al. 1989[9]	4	4 (100%)	22*
Gledhill and Dixon 1998[25]	9	9 (100%)	12–120
Burroughs et al. 1998[26]	8	8 (100%)	51*
Gelb and Finkelstein 1974[23]	1	1 (100%)	Not provided
Naouri et al. 1992[24]	3	3 (100%)	36*
Goldstein et al. 2000[27]	25	23 (92*)	91*
Total	50	48 (96%)	Not applicable

While there are characteristic clinical, endoscopic, and radiological features of CD, the diagnosis is usually only fully established by pathological examination. The three pathological hallmarks of CD are transmural inflammation, epithelioid cell granulomata, and fissuring or fistula. While biopsies may strongly suggest the diagnosis, a definitive diagnosis of CD is often made only at the time of intestinal resection. It is clear from several papers describing the association of sigmoid CD and diverticulosis that the diagnosis was indeed made at the time of resection[6,7,9]. All three pathological hallmarks of CD may be caused by complicated diverticular disease with diverticulitis and peridiverticulitis alone. Even granulomas and crypt abscesses in the mucosa may accompany the luminal mucosal inflammatory response that occurs in diverticular disease (Table 3).

Many older patients have coexistent atheromatous disease, leading to relative ischaemia of the colon. The combination of this and changes in bacterial flora, secondary to stasis secondary within the diverticula can be responsible for the Crohn-like inflammatory response in the sigmoid colon[8].

The prognosis of patients with a suggested coexistence of CD and diverticular disease in the rectosigmoid and no evidence of CD elsewhere in the gastrointestinal tract seems remarkably good[6,7,9] (Figure 3). This suggests

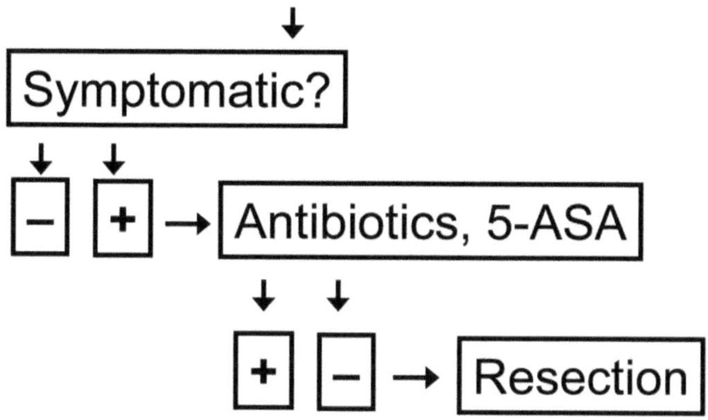

Figure 3 Treatment: diverticular disease without prior Crohn's disease

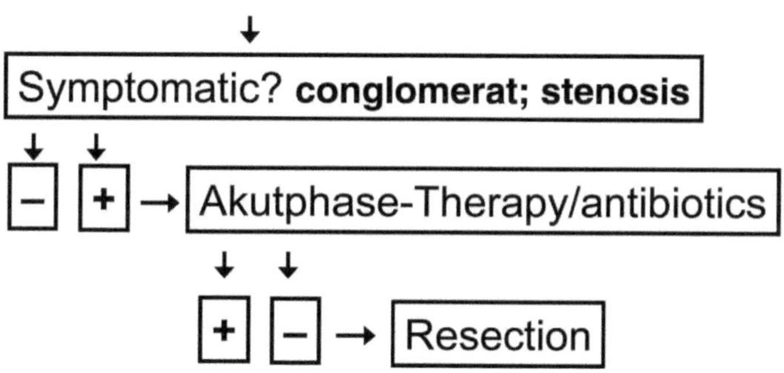

Figure 4 Treatment: diverticular disease and prior or concurrent Crohn's disease

that some of these cases simply represent a complicated diverticulosis with pathological mimicry of CD (Table 3). Therefore the entire gastrointestinal tract should be investigated in cases in which apparent CD complicates diverticular disease of the sigmoid colon, and the therapy should be adapted (Figure 4).

CONCLUSIONS

Diverticular disease may be associated with complex inflammatory characteristics that may closely mimic IBD. Clinical evidence would suggest that the coexistence of diverticulosis and CD is commoner than the prevalence of either would suggest; but the association may be exaggerated. The situation is just as uncertain with UC, because of mimicry of that disease by luminal inflammation in diverticular disease. In some patients the latter may represent a specific form of inflammatory bowel disease, which responds well to treatment that is effective in IBD. Occasional cases of diverticular colitis suggest a relationship between diverticular colitis and UC, which may provide insights into the pathogenesis of UC[10].

References

1. Manousos ON, Truelove SC, Lumsden K. Prevalence of colonic diverticulosis in the general population of Oxford area. Br Med J. 1967;3:762–3.
2. Calkins BM, Mendeloff AI. The epidemiology of idiopathic inflammatory bowel disease. In: Kirsner JB, Shorter RG, editors. Inflammatory Bowel Disease. Baltimore: Williams & Wilkins, 1995:31–68.
3. Shapiro PA, Peppercorn MA, Antonioli DA, Joffe N, Goldman H. Crohn's disease in the elderly. Am J Gastroenterol. 1981;76:132–7.
4. Tchircow G, Lavery IC, Fazio VW. Crohn's disease in the elderly. Dis Colon Rectum. 1983; 26:177–81.
5. Carr N, Schofield PF. Inflammatory bowel disease in the older patient. Br J Surg. 1982; 69:223–5.
6. Berman IR, Corman ML, Coller JA, Veidenheimer MC. Late onset Crohn's disease in patients with colonic diverticular disease. Dis Colon Rectum. 1979;22:524–9.
7. Schmidt GT, Lennard-Jones JE, Morson BC, Young AC. Crohn's disease of the colon and its distinction from diverticulitis. Gut. 1968;9:7–16.
8. Meyers MA, Alonso DR, Morson BC, Bartram C. Pathogenesis of diverticulitis complicating granulomatous colitis. Gastroenterology. 1978;74:24–31.
9. McCue J, Coppen MJ, Rasbridge SA, Lock MR. Coexistent Crohn's disease and sigmoid diverticulosis. Postgrad Med J. 1989;65:636–9.
10. Shepherd NA. Pathological mimics of chronic inflammatory bowel disease. J Clin Pathol. 1991;44:726–33.
11. Gore S, Shepherd NA, Wilkinson SP. Endoscopic crescentic fold disease of the sigmoid colon: the clinical and histopathological spectrum of a distinctive endoscopic appearance. Int J Colorect Dis. 1992;7:76–81.
12. Peppercorn MA. Drug-responsive chronic segmental colitis associated with diverticular: a clinical syndrome in the elderly. Am J Gastroenterol. 1992;87:609–12.
13. Makapugay LM, Dean PJ. Diverticular disease-associated chronic colitis. Am J Surg Pathol. 1996;20:94–102.
14. Hart J, Baert F, Hanauer S. Sigmoiditis: a clinical syndrome with a spectrum of pathological features, including a distinctive form of IBD. Mod Pathol. 1995;8:62A
15. Imperiali G, Meucci G, Alvisi C et al. Segmental colitis associated with divertcular: a prospective study. Am J Gastroenterol. 2000;95:1014–16.
16. Sladen GE, Filipe MI. Is segmental colitis a complication of diverticular disease? Dis Colon Rectum. 1984;27:513–14.
17. Cawthorn SJ, Gibbs NM, Marks GG. Segmental colitis: a new complication of diverticular colitis. Gut. 1983;24:A500.
18. Rhodes J, Rose J. Crohn's disease in the elderly. Br Med J. 1985;291:1149–50.
19. Ludeman L, Shepherd NA. What is diverticular colitis? Pathology. 2002;34:568–72.
20. Polit SA. Chronic segmental colitis in association with diverticolosis: a clinical syndrome in the elderly? J Am Geriatr Soc. 1993;41:1155–6.

21. van Rosendaal GM, Andersen MA. Segmental colitis complicating diverticular disease. Can J Gastroenterol. 1996;10:361–4.
22. Pereira MC. Diverticular disease-associated colitis: progression to severe chronic ulcerative colitis after sigmoid surgery. Gastrointest Endosc. 1998;48:520–3.
23. Gelb AM, Finkelstein WE. Differential diagnosis of diverticulitis and granulomatous colitis. Exacerbation of granulomatous colitis after sigmoid resection. Am J Gastroenterol. 1974;62:9–15.
24. Naouri A, Maroun J, Tissot E. Diverticulosis and Crohn's disease of the sigmoid. Ann Chir. 1992;46:67–70.
25. Gledhill A, Dixon MP. Crohn's-like reaction in diverticular disease. Gut. 1998;42:392–5.
26. Burroughs SH, Bowrey DJ, Morris-Stiff GJ, Williams GT. Granulomatous inflammation of sigmoid diverticulitis: two diseases or one? Histopathology. 1998;33:349–53.
27. Goldstein NS, Leon-Armin C, Mani A. Crohn's colitis-like changes in sigmoid diverticulitis specimens is usually an idiosyncratic inflammatory response to the diverticulosis rather than Crohn's colitis. Am J Surg Pathol. 2000;24:668–75.

Section V
Indications and controversies in imaging techniques

Chair: P. MARTEAU and S. POST

10
Colonoscopy in acute diverticulitis*

S. BAR-MEIR, A. LAHAT and I. SAKHNINI

Acute colonic diverticulitis is an inflammatory process that complicates diverticular disease. When clinical symptoms are present the inflammation is already transmural and may extend to the adjacent pericolonic fat and surrounding organs. Acute diverticulitis is regarded as representing a sealed perforation of the colonic wall. The diagnosis of acute colonic diverticulitis is based on the clinical presentation and on computed tomography (CT) scanning[1–4].

Occasionally, however, an adenocarcinoma of the colon may mimic both the clinical presentation and the CT appearance of acute diverticulitis. In these patients only colonoscopy is of diagnostic value. However, common practice after an acute diverticulitis event is to postpone colonoscopy for a period of 6 weeks in order to prevent the conversion of a sealed perforation into a free one[5–9].

The clinical relevance of colonoscopy during the acute stage of diverticulitis has not been studied. We therefore studied the effect of early colonoscopy on the outcome of patients with acute colonic diverticulitis. The following study was published in *Endoscopy*[10].

Consecutive patients hospitalized for acute left lower abdominal pain and fever, in whom acute diverticulitis was suspected, were evaluated prospectively. All patients underwent an abdominal CT, and only patients with findings compatible with a diagnosis of acute diverticulitis were included in the study. The CT criteria for acute diverticulitis included the presence of a colonic diverticulum, colonic wall thickening at the location of the diverticulum, and pericolonic fat infiltration. In the first part of the study, patients with CT findings of extracolonic air or fluid adjacent to a diverticulum were excluded. During the second phase of the study only patients with free colonic perforation, i.e. free intraperitoneal air, were excluded. Patients who had had a colonoscopy within 1 year before the current episode of acute diverticulitis

* Part of this chapter was previously published in Endoscopy 2004;36:504–8.

were also excluded, as additional colonoscopy was considered unnecessary. All patients were hospitalized and treated with intravenous antibiotics. A complete colonoscopy was performed at a later time during their hospitalization, preferably on the day of discharge. Bowel cleansing was carried out with an oral phosphosoda preparation (Soffodex, Dexxon, Hadera, Israel) given orally 1 day before the procedure. The colonoscopies were carried out by three endoscopists with at least 10 years of experience each, with the patients receiving conscious sedation with intravenous midazolam (Midolam, Rafa Laboratories Ltd, Jerusalem, Israel) 2.5–5.0 mg and pethidine (Dolestine, Biogal, Hungary) 50 mg. The patients remained in hospital for at least an additional 6 h and were discharged thereafter if no symptoms suggestive of perforation had developed. All patients were contacted by telephone 1 and 3 days after the procedure and were asked about the presence of findings suggestive of perforation, such as abdominal pain and fever. The study was approved by the local ethics committee, and all of the patients provided informed consent.

A total of 122 patients with acute diverticulitis were admitted to the Chaim Sheba Medical Center, Tel Hashomer, Israel, between July 2000 and January 2003. Four patients had undergone colonoscopy during the previous year and were therefore not offered another examination. Another 11 patients declined to participate in the study. The remaining 107 patients (47 men, 60 women; median age 63 years, range 30–89 years) agreed to have colonoscopy and were included in the study). Ninety patients were experiencing acute diverticulitis for the first time and 17 for the second time. During the first phase of the study 49 patients agreed to have colonoscopy. Ten of these patients were excluded because of either peridiverticular air (nine patients) or peridiverticular fluid (one patient). The remaining 39 patients underwent colonoscopy.

During the second phase of the study 58 patients agreed to have colonoscopy. Four patients were excluded because of the presence of free intraperitoneal air on the CT scan and clinical symptoms of intestinal perforation. These four patients underwent surgery; the diagnosis was confirmed and the sigmoid colon was resected. The remaining 54 patients underwent colonoscopy, six of whom had pericolonic air or fluid. Colonoscopy was carried out 4–12 days after admission (median 5.8 days). Complete colonoscopy with caecal intubation was achieved in 75 patients. The reasons for failed caecal intubation were colonic stricture at the site of the diverticulitis (10 patients), pain (five patients), malignant obstruction (one patient), and poor colonic preparation (two patients). At colonoscopy, diverticula were seen in all except four patients. Barium enema examinations were carried out at a later stage in three of these four patients, revealing diverticula in two and a normal colon in the third. The fourth patient refused to have a barium enema. There was no explanation for the clinical presentation of diverticulitis in the patient who had no evidence of a diverticulum at either colonoscopy or barium enema. The patient with a malignant obstruction was a 55-year-old man. He had presented at another hospital 2 months earlier with clinical findings of acute diverticulitis. His condition had improved with conservative therapy, and he was recommended to undergo colonoscopy 6 weeks later. He did not appear for the checkup examination and was admitted to our hospital with a similar presentation suggestive of acute diverticulitis. A colonoscopy was carried out, and an obstructive, malignant-looking mass was detected in the sigmoid colon. The histological findings showed that it was an adenocarcinoma. Surgery was carried out, and the patient was discharged 10 days later.

Additional findings on colonoscopy included the presence of 11 polyps in nine patients. The polyps were located in the rectum ($n = 2$), descending colon ($n = 4$), and ascending colon ($n = 5$). One of the patients had two polyps located in the rectum and caecum, another patient had two polyps located in the ascending and descending colon. The size of the 11 polyps varied from 10 to 20 mm. All of the polyps were resected uneventfully. Pathology demonstrated tubular adenoma in nine cases, tubulovillous adenoma in one case, and tubulovillous adenoma with infiltrating adenocarcinoma in another. The resection margins for the malignant polyp were free of carcinoma. The latter patient was an elderly patient who might otherwise not have attended for a later scheduled colonoscopy.

All of the patients except one underwent colonoscopy with no complications. One patient developed a free perforation of the sigmoid colon after the colonoscopy; she was an 88-year-old woman in whom the initial CT had shown air located adjacent to the wall of a diverticulum. She was treated with intravenous antibiotics, and showed marked clinical improvement. A complete colonoscopy was performed on hospital day 9. Several hours later her abdomen became distended and free air was detected on a plain abdominal radiograph. Surgery was carried out, and a perforation of the sigmoid colon was identified. A Hartmann operation was carried out, and the patient was discharged 2 weeks later.

In one patient the colonoscopy appeared to be of major therapeutic value. This was a 73-year-old woman in whom symptoms of acute diverticulitis continued for 10 days without improvement. She was treated in hospital using broad-spectrum antibiotics, but with no response. She underwent colonoscopy on hospital day 10, and a small chicken bone trapped in a diverticulum was identified. There was a purulent discharge from the diverticulum. After the bone had been removed the patient's condition improved and she was discharged 1 day later.

The caecum was not reached during the first colonoscopy in 18 patients. A second colonoscopy 6 weeks later was carried out successfully in 16. The other two patients underwent surgery, due to obstructing adenocarcinoma of the sigmoid colon in one case and recurrent episodes of diverticulitis in the other.

This study provides a basis for assessing the level of risk involved and the information capable of being provided when colonoscopy is carried out by an experienced endoscopist in a patient with acute diverticulitis. This type of procedure is associated with a lower rate of caecal intubation and probably a higher risk of perforation, but it may alter the outcome in patients with a refractory course.

Persently we are in the midst of a prospective randomized control trial in which patients who are being hospitalized because of acute diverticulitis are being randomized into either immediate colonoscopy during hospitalization or 6 weeks later. Patients with either pericolic air or free perforation are being excluded. Also excluded are patients who underwent colonoscopy within the last year.

Sixty-two patients were randomized, 32 for an immediate colonoscopy and 30 for a delayed procedure. Only one tubular adenomatous polyp was identified among the patients who underwent the colonoscopy during their hospitalization. Of the 30 patients who were randomized for a delayed colonoscopy, seven did not show up for the examination. Three patients were found to have polyps, tubular and villous tubular adenoma. None of the 62 patients had cancer and in none of the patients had a complication occurred. In four patients of the immediate colonoscopy group, and in three of the delayed group, the colonoscope cuold not reach the caecum.

If the results of our ongoing study remain the same with a larger number of patients, we will recommend the following: (a) CT scan in acute diverticulitis is sufficient to exclude the presence of colorectal cancer; (b) routine colonoscopy is not advocated; (c) colonoscopy should be reserved only for acute diverticulitis patients with a refractory course; (d) presence of pericolic air on CT may carry an increased risk for colonoscopy during the acute phase; (e) colonoscopy in acute diverticulitis is feasible, but seldom necessary.

References

1. Cho KC, Morehouse HT, Alterman DD, Thornhill BA. Sigmoid diverticulitis: diagnostic role of CT – comparison with barium enema studies. Radiology. 1990;176:111–15.
2. Rao PM. CT of diverticulitis and alternative conditions. Semin Ultrasound CT MR. 1999;20:86–93.
3. Hulnick DH, Megibow AJ, Balthazar EJ et al. Computed tomography in the evaluation of diverticulitis. Radiology. 1984;152:491–5.
4. Hachigian MP, Honickman S, Eisenstat TE et al. Computed tomography in the initial management of acute left-sided diverticulitis. Dis Colon Rectum. 1992;35:1123–9.
5. Almy TP, Howell DA. Medical progress. diverticular disease of the colon. N Engl J Med. 1980;302:324–31.
6. Penfold JC. Perforation of the colon complicating colonoscopy: report of a case. Dis Colon Rectum. 1975;18:626–7.
7. Forde KA. Colonoscopy in complicated diverticular disease. Gastrointest Endosc. 1977;23:192–3.
8. Dean AC, Newell JP. Colonoscopy in the differential diagnosis of carcinoma from diverticulitis of the sigmoid colon. Br J Surg. 1973;60:633–5.
9. Panish JF. Limitations and complications of colonoscopy. Gastrointest Endosc. 1980;26:20S–1.
10. Sakhnini E, Lahat A, Melzer E et al. Early colonoscopy in patients with acute diverticulitis: results of a prospective pilot study. Endoscopy. 2004;36:504–7.

11 Sonography in diverticular disease

S. SCHANZ

Ultrasound (US) is carried out as a primary diagnostic method in most cases of abdominal pain. The reasons are broad availability, at least in Germany and central Europe, and the possibility of immediate application even in emergency rooms at the admission of the patient. Ultrasound of the abdomen is realized by both internists and surgeons. Examination of the entire colon should be an integral part of any abdominal scanning, although it requires special experience in US of the bowel. It is possible to image most parts of the large bowel and unsuspected pathology may be detected. In various clinical situations an examination targeted at the colon may produce valuable information. However, is there really a role for US in diverticular disease? When studying current reviews in journals of international repute one might come to the conclusion that this technique has not become standard practice[1,2]. Regarding the best imaging technique for unclear abdominal conditions there are a few criteria for an ideal examination method. There must be a broad availability at low cost. The technique should have no side-effects, must be easy to learn and handle and should be repeatable at any time. US fulfils most of these criteria.

US is useful to describe normal bowel wall and also pathological changes. With the introduction of high-frequency probes with a range from 5 to 10 MHz and better US machines in recent years it has become much easier to differentiate normal small bowel and colon from other structures. Colour and power Doppler equipment for vascular detection to graduate inflammation or to identify necrosis is helpful. As in any other technique the examiner should have experience in sonography of the bowel. The normal intestinal wall stratifies five layers alternating hypoechoic and hyperechoic layer which cover all parts of the intestine (Figure 1).

Clear recognition of both walls depends on the colonic content and condition of the bowel. If the colon is empty, both walls may be opposed with graduated compression so that a central reflection from the mucosal surface is not seen, or is seen only with difficulty. Semi-solid residues are moderately reflective. Gas causes a major reverberation echo, but the colonic wall next to the transducer may still be visible (Figure 2). Abdominal US is sometimes limited by overlying gas that obscures the diseased segment, and may produce false-negative results. This problem is accentuated by obesity or a localized ileus in the small bowel next to the acute process.

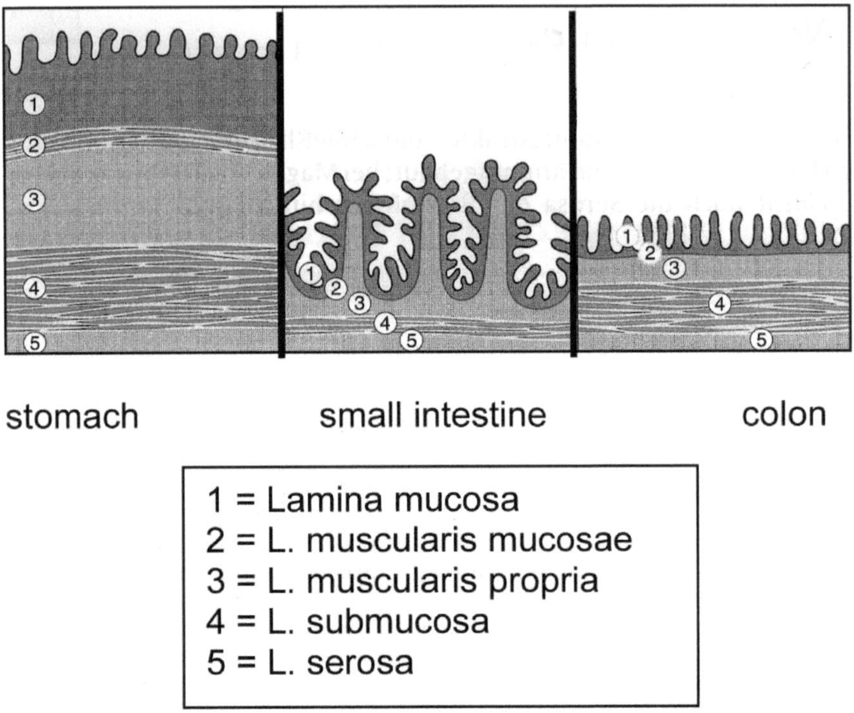

Figure 1 Five sonographic layers of the intestine

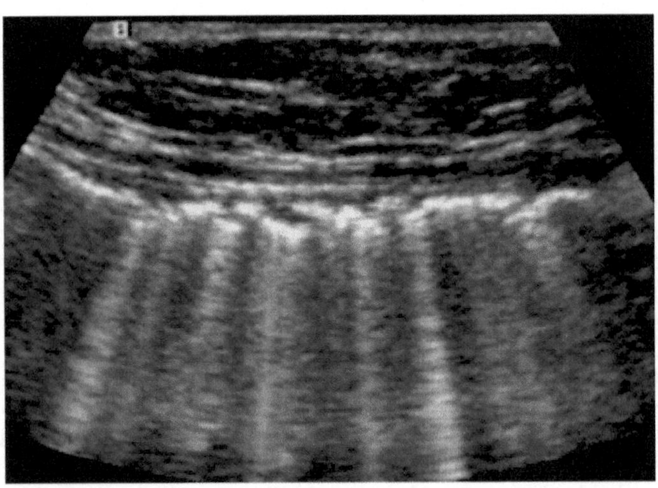

Figure 2 Normal colon with gas

In most cases, however, the colonic wall, especially that of the sigmoid colon, can be recognized. The wall in the left-sided colon measures 3–4 mm in thickness. Diverticular disease is characterized by longitudinal muscle contraction in the sigmoid colon resulting in wall thickening and interdigitating folds of the muscle. Intra- and extramural diverticula can be visualized as hyperechoic, bright foci with varying degrees of acoustic shadowing representing air (Figure 3).

Regarding diverticulosis there is one prospective study from Hollerweger et al.[3] from Austria. They investigated the ability of sonography compared with endoscopy to diagnose diverticulosis, and demonstrated the typical appearance of normal diverticula. These were assessed for number, diameter, echogenicity and wall thickness. Sonography detected 28 of 33 patients with endoscopically proven diverticula although US on average could demonstrate less diverticula per patient than endoscopy. The sigmoid colon was found in all cases; all diverticula except one were hyperechoic. The authors, and this is also my personal experience, concluded that US can diagnose diverticulosis in most cases. In complicated diverticular disease, the clinically more relevant problem, US can determine pathological changes with the same criteria used in computed tomography (CT): colonic wall thickening, pericolic and peridiverticular inflammation. An inflamed diverticulum, a so-called 'dome sign', is characterized by its location in the centre of a pericolic inflammation which has a sensitivity of 80% for the diagnosis of diverticulitis[4] (Figure 4). The investigator may note additional clinical signs such as tenderness or pain on compression of the involved area, which is emphasized by Schwerk et al.[5] (Table 1).

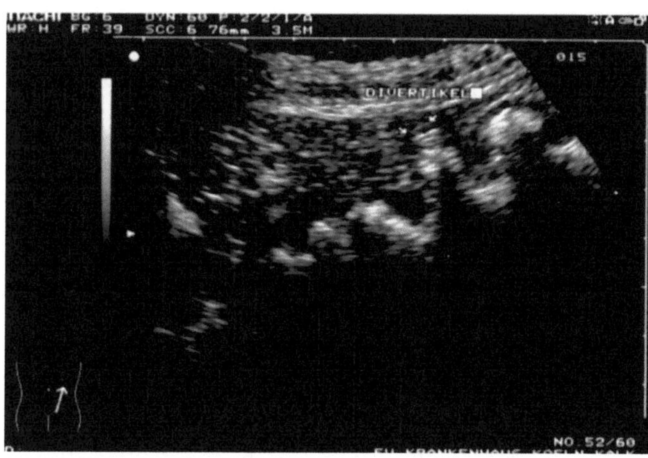

Figure 3 Longitudinal sectioning of the sigmoid colon with diverticula

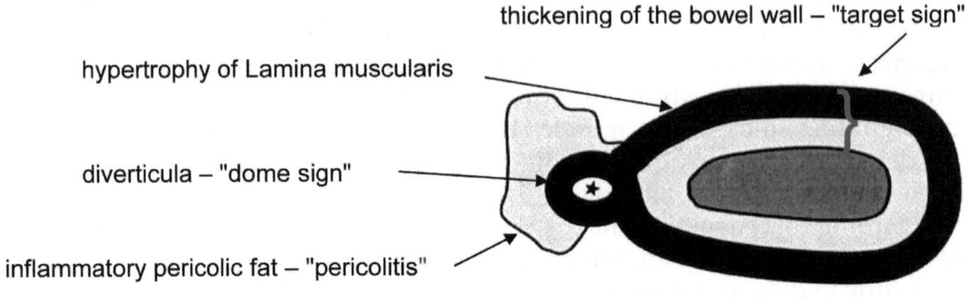

Figure 4 Sonographic appearance in acute diverticulitis

Table 1 Sonographic citeria in acute diverticulitis

Colonic wall >5 mm
Target/pseudokidney sign
Diverticulum ('dome sign')
Pain/tenderness on compression of the involved area
Peridiverticulitis
Intramural/peridiverticular abscess
Colovesicle fistula

The accuracy of US in diverticulitis is documented since 1985 by Parekular et al[5]. Since then the effectiveness of US has been recognized in several prospective studies[6–8] (Table 2). The same sonographic criteria can be applied in right-sided diverticulitis of the caecum and ascending colon with excellent sensitivity and specificity[9,10].

Similar to CT, US is capable of evaluating the transmural involvement of the inflammation. Figures 5a–d demonstrate hypoechoic thickening of the wall of the involved segment of the colon greater than 5 mm with a central echogenic focus. A rigid zone of increased echogenicity adjacent to the colon wall represents omental or pericolic fat encasing the inflammatory process. Extramural diverticula are visualized as hypoechoic outpouchings of the inflamed wall, often with hyperechoic foci representing air or residue within the lumen of the diverticulum.

Especially in the ill patient the initial use of US may obviate the need for CT with intraluminal and intravenous contrast in the acute stage. In addition US is highly sensitive in detecting complications of diverticular disease[6–8,11,12]. Despite these favourable results using US in diverticular disease there is ongoing discussion regarding the diagnostic limitations related to operator dependence compared with CT, in which subjective interpretation seems to be less problematic. However, this argument should be used for any examination technique and even for clinical examination. So-called limited operator expertise is also valid for CT.

Table 2 Ultrasound studies in diverticular disease

Reference	*n*	*Sensitivity (%)*	*Specificity (%)*
Federman 1989[18]	23	96	98
Verbanck et al. 1989[11]	123	85	80
Wilson and Toi 1990[12]	54	85	–
Wada et al. 1990[19]	18*	100	100
Schwerk et al. 1992[8]	52	98	98
Schwerk et al. 1993[20]	74	99	97
Zielke et al. 1997[21]	74	84	93
Estaban Hernandez et al. 1998[22]	19	95	100
Pisanu et al. 2000[23]	22	95	91
Hollerweger et al. 2001[15]	102	77	99
Chou et al. 2001[10]	23*	91	100
Alberti et al. 2002[24]	51	91	100
Moll et al. 2002[25]	247	76	97
Ripollés et al. 2003[26]	203	94	98
Farag Soliman et al. 2004[13]	63	97	97
Total	1148	91	96

*Right-sided diverticulitis

In some of the demonstrated studies it is mentioned that examinations were performed mostly by residents on duty instead of expert sonographers, depending on the time of the request for exploration. The recently published prospective study by Farag-Soliman and co-workers[13] revealed the important role of US in the diagnostic work-up of surgeons. Sixty-three patients with clinical suspicion of diverticulitis were examined initially by US followed by CT. Sensitivity and specificity for both techniques was 97%. However, US has some limitations in assessing large and complex abscesses (Figure 6) or in inflammation of the distal sigmoid deep in the pelvis, which is sometimes barely accessible. Recently, some institutions have employed transrectal sonography to complement transabdominal sonography[14].

In addition, there is some overlap with other inflammatory diseases that can mimic diverticulitis, e.g. Crohn's disease, and ischaemic or infectious colitis with or without benign diverticulosis. In these cases, or if there is any discrepancy between clinical and sonographic findings, the experienced clinician would proceed to other diagnostic procedures, especially CT. Another important differential diagnosis for diverticulitis is epiploic appendagitis characterized by hyperechoic pericolic fat[15]. However, the absence of bowel wall thickening and colour Doppler signals in the altered pericolic fat in epiploic appendagitis are criteria for differentiation.

Large bowel obstructions can sometimes be seen within an acute episode of inflammation. but usually reflect repeated prior episodes of diverticulitis with stricture formation. However, both CT and US have difficulties in differentiating a diverticular stricture from a colon cancer (Figure 7).

Involved segments over 10 cm, as well as a lack of a shoulder formation within the lumen are more suggestive of diverticulitis[16]. After the acute phase it is currently considered that the colon should be evaluated by a follow-up colonoscopy (Table 3).

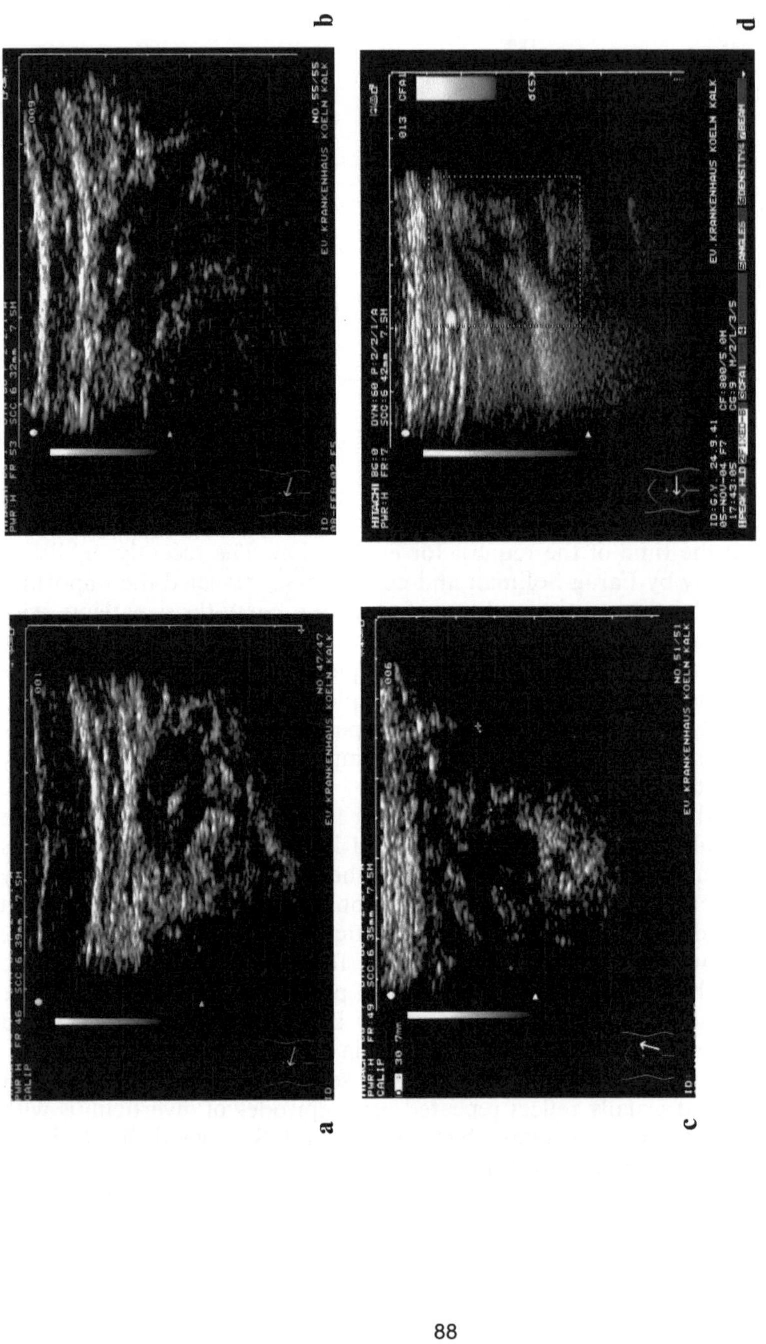

Figure 5 Examples of acute (peri-)diverticulitis. (The black arrow in panel (**d**) shows a large diverticulum)

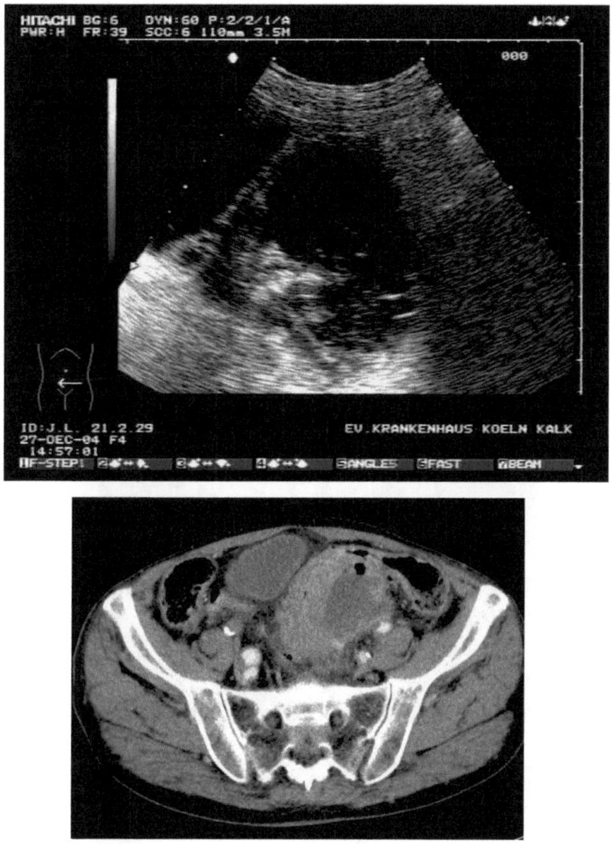

Figure 6 Paravesical abscess due to acute diverticulitis of the sigmoid colon (with corresponding CT)

Nevertheless, the above-mentioned favourable results support the use of US as initial imaging in patients referred for lower quadrant or pelvis pain, including patients with clinical suspicion of acute diverticulitis. The costs are minimal compared to the more elaborate CT. There are no procedure-related side-effects. and US can be repeated at any time as an ideal follow-up method. If follow-up sonography is performed, the inflamed diverticula may change their sonographic appearance[17]. Spontaneous evacuation of pus or a faecalith into the colonic lumen may occur. The echogenicity of diverticula can change with the decrease of swelling and wall thickening, resulting in various amounts of gas in the lumen of the diverticula with varying acoustic shadowing. Mostly, the attending physician who plans the treatment is also the examiner, which is an additional valuable argument in favour of US. The doctor who is already familiar with the patients' history, physical findings and laboratory tests applies US to reach a diagnostic hypothesis. The background of abnormal findings

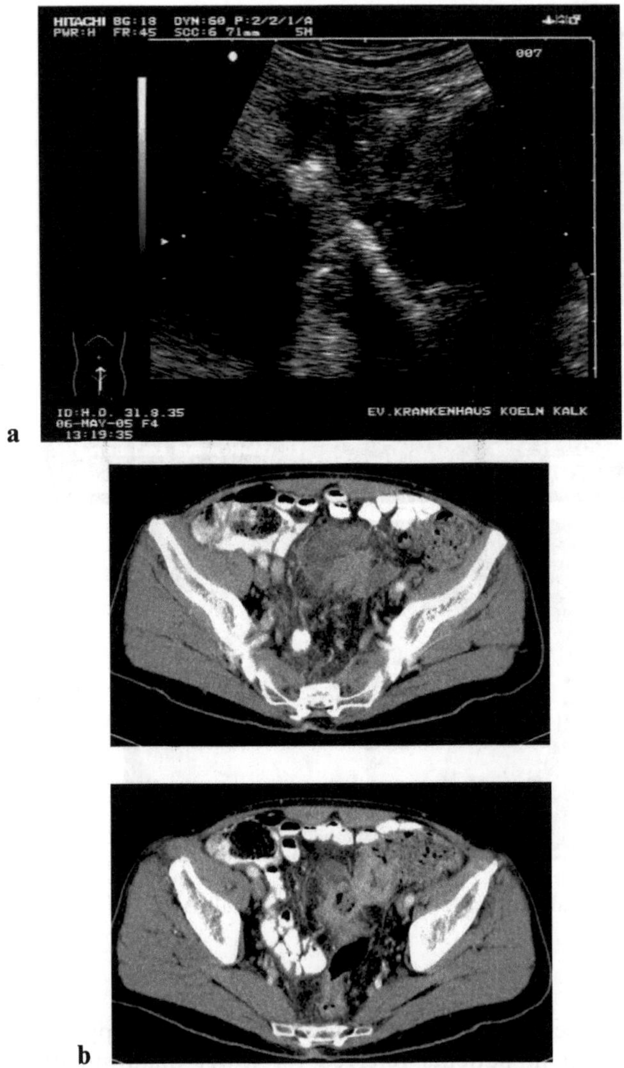

Figure 7 Perforated carcinoma of the sigmoid: (a) white arrow: perforation site with gas, white pointed arrow: hypoechoic abscess formation; (b) corresponding CT sections

allows the doctor an immediate plausibility control, if the conclusion is the most probable. If there is a major doubt, he/she would go to the next step and proceed to cross-sectional imaging.

To conclude, US, as an initial imaging technique, is sufficient in 80–90% of patients with suspected diverticulitis, CT should be reserved for doubtful cases or discrepant clinical evolutions (Table 4).

Table 3 Limitations of US in diverticular disease

Large and complex abscess
Distal sigmoid involvement
Overlap between colonic cancer and other inflammatory diseases

Table 4 Advantages of US in diverticular disease

Wide availability
Diagnostic method with sufficient sensitivity
Low cost
No iodinated contrast material
No side-effects (radiation, hyperthyroidism, renal failure)
Examiner = attending physician

With the coming of the DRG (Diagnostic Related Groups) era, this will emphasize the economic role of sonography, the necessity for appropriate coding and the need for more sonographic training. Only high quality will increase the acceptance of US as an important diagnostic tool.

References

1. Ferzoco LB, Raptopoulos V, Silen W. Acute diverticulitis. N Engl J Med. 1998;338:1521–6.
2. Stollman N, Raskin JB. Diverticular disease of the colon. Lancet. 2004;363:631–9.
3. Hollerweger A, Macheiner P, Hübner E, Brunner W, Gritzmann N. Colonic diverticulosis: a comparison between sonography and endoscopy. Ultraschall Med. 2002;23:41–6.
4. Kori T, Nemoto M, Maeda M et al. Sonographic features of acute coloniic diverticulitis: the 'dome sign'. J Clin Ultrasound. 2000;28:340–64.
5. Schwerk WB, Wichtrup B, Rothmund M, Ruschoff J. Ultrasonography in the diagnosis of acute appendicitis: a prospective study. Gastroenterology. 1989;97:630–9.
6. Parekular SG. Sonography of colonic diverticulitis. J Ultrasound Med. 1985;4:659–66.
7. Pradel JA, Adell JF, Taoural P, Djafori M, Mounin-Delhom E, Bruel JM. Acute colonic diverticulitis: a prospective comparative evaluation with US and CT. Radiol. 1997;205:503–12.
8. Schwerk WB, Schwarz S, Rothmund M. Sonography in acute colonic diverticulitis. A prospective study. Dis Colon Rectum. 1992;35:1077–84.
9. Wada M, Kikuchi Y, Doy M. Uncomplicated acute diverticulitis of the caecum and ascending colon: sonographic findings in 18 patients. Am J Roentgenol. 1990;155:283–7.
10. Chou YH, Chiou HJ, Chen JD et al. Sonography of acute right side colonic diverticulitis. Am J Surg. 2001;181:122–7.
11. Verbanck J, Lambrecht S, Rutgeerts L et al. Can sonography diagnose acute colonic diverticulitis in patients with acute intestinal inflammation? A prospective study. J Clin Ultrasound. 1989;17:661–6.
12. Wilson SR, Toi A. The value of sonography in the diagnosis of acute diverticulitis of the colon. Am J Roentgenol. 1990;154:1199–202.
13. Farag Soliman M, Wüstner M, Sturm J et al. Primary diagnostics of acute diverticulitis of the the sigmoid. Sonography versus computed tomography: a prospective study. Ultraschall Med. 2004;25:342–7.
14. Hollerweger A, Rettenbacher T, Macheiner P, Brunner W, Gritzmann N. Sigmoid diverticulitis: value of transrectal sonography in addition to transabdominal sonography. Am J Roentgenol. 2000;175:1155–60.

15. Hollerweger A, Macheiner P, Rettenbacher T, Brunner W, Gritzmann N. Colonic diverticulitis: diagnostic value and appearance of inflamed diverticula – sonographic evaluation. Eur Radiol. 2001;11:1956–63.
16. Chintapalli KN, Chopra S, Ghiatas AA, Esola CC, Fields SF, Dodd GD. Diverticulitis versus colon cancer: differentiation with helical CT findings. Radiology. 1999;210:429–35.
17. Oudenhoven LFIJ, Koumans RKJ, Puylaert JBCM. Right colonic diverticulitis: US and CT findings: new insights about frequency and natural history. Radiology. 1998;208:611–18.
18. Federmann G. Sonographie in der Diagnostik der akuten Divertikulitis. Der Chirurg. 1989;60:415–18.
19. Wada M, Kikuchi Y, Doy M. Uncomplicated acute diverticulitis of the cecum and the ascending colon: sonographic findings in 18 patients. Am J Roentgenol. 1990;155:283–7.
20. Schwerk WB, Schwarz S, Rothmund M, Arnold R. Colon diverticulitis: imaging diagnosis with ultrasound – a prospective study. Z Gastroenterol. 1993;31:294–300.
21. Zielke A, Hasse C, Nies C et al. Prospective evaluation of ultrasonography in acute colonic diverticulitis. Br J Surg. 1997;84:383–8.
22. Esteban Hernandez JM, Maldonado Blanco L, Leon Guijarro JL, Pascual Moreno I, Nogues Pelayo E. Value of ultrasonography as the initial diagnostic method in acute sigmoid diverticulitis. Gastroenterol Hepatol. 1998;21:423–6.
23. Pisanu A, Floris G, Secci L, Uccheddu A. Ultrasonography of acute diverticulitis. Effect on surgical treatment. G Chir. 2000;21:297–302.
24. Alberti A, Dattola P, Parisi A, Maccarone P, Basile M. Role of ultrasonographic imaging in the surgical management of acute diverticulitis of the colon. Chir Ital. 2002;54:71–5.
25. Moll R, Mittelkotter U, Reith HB, Schindler G, Thiede A. Which imaging in case of sigmoid diverticulitis? The value of ultrasound in comparison to the well-established modalities like contrast enema and helical computer tomography. Zentralbl Chir. 2002;127:297–301.
26. Ripollés T, Agramunt M, Martínez MJ, Costa S, Gómez-Abril SA, Richart J. The role of ultrasound in the diagnosis, management and evolutive prognosis of acute left-sided colonic diverticulitis: a review of 208 cases. Eur Radiol. 2003;13:2587–95.

12 Diverticular disease: abdominal radiography, contrast enema, computed tomography, magnetic resonance imaging

S. FEUERBACH

INTRODUCTION

Diverticular disease is a common entity. This acquired abnormality occurs in 85% in the sigmoid colon, and most patients will remain entirely asymptomatic. Thus, the incidental identification of diverticulosis by contrast enema, colonoscopy, ultrasound, computed tomography or magnetic resonance imaging does not require any further diagnostic evaluation[1]. In the following, the role of abdominal radiographs, contrast enema, computed tomography (CT) and magnetic resonance imaging (MRI) in the diagnosis and staging of diverticulitis is reviewed.

ABDOMINAL RADIOGRAPHY

Abdominal radiography has traditionally been considered an essential part of the work-up in patients with acute abdominal pain, although the results are often non-specific. In a recent study CT was compared with abdominal plain films in 188 patients who underwent both imaging modalities[2]. Only 10% of the radiographs were abnormal, and the sensitivity for the specific diagnosis of appendicitis, pyelonephritis, pancreatitis and diverticulitis was 0%! Due to the lack of impact on further diagnostic evaluation or therapy, abdominal plain films can no longer be recommended as a routine examination in patients with the typical clinical symptoms of diverticulitis.

BARIUM ENEMA

Before the CT and ultrasound era barium enema was considered the standard examination for diverticulitis. This examination provides information on the number and location of diverticula with lumen stenosis. The typical signs of diverticulitis in barium enemas are bowel wall oedema, spasm, intramural fistulas and, in the case of perforation, contrast extravasation and free air bubbles (Figure 1). The study of Ambrosetti et al.[3] compares the performance of a water-soluble contrast enema with that of CT in 420 patients with clinically suspected left colonic diverticulitis. The performance of CT was significantly superior to contrast enema in terms of sensitivity (98% vs 92%), which was calculated from patients who had histologically proven diverticulitis. Moreover, only 20 (29%) of 69 patients with associated abscesses, verified by CT, had indirect signs of these complications on contrast enema[3]. This demonstrates the disadvantages of contrast enemas compared to all cross-sectional imaging techniques: diverticulitis is mainly an extraluminal process, which is identified using CT or ultrasound, but not or only with indirect signs by contrast enemas. Contrast enema is no longer a standard technique, but a reliable alternative modality, if CT and ultrasound are not available. If performed, only water-soluble contrast medium is recommended[4].

COMPUTED TOMOGRAPHY

Even though ultrasound and CT have similar sensitivity and specificity[5], in many institutions CT is the method of choice, because of its ability to image extraluminal disease as well as its therapeutic potential in abscess drainage. Compared to ultrasound, CT is an operator-independent examination with an excellent documentation, which is easily understood by all – gastroenterologists, surgeons and radiologists.

The typical CT findings in diverticulitis are: segmental wall thickening; lumen narrowing; fat stranding, fascial thickening; diverticula, 'arrowhead sign'; abscesses; perforation with contrast medium extravasation and/or extraluminal air (Figures 2 and 3).

Kircher et al.[6] determined the frequency, sensitivity and specificity of these individual signs of diverticulitis using helical CT with rectally administered contrast material. The design of the study was a retrospective analysis of the prospective interpretation. CT interpretations were correlated with patients' clinical courses and surgical findings. The two most frequent signs of diverticulitis were bowel wall thickening in 96% and fat stranding in 95%. Less frequent, but highly specific signs were fascial thickening (50%), free fluid (45%), inflamed diverticula (43%) and free air (30%) (Table 1).

Because diverticulitis occurs predominantly in older people, the differentiation between diverticulitis and colon cancer is very important. Moreover, both entities can be present in the same patient. Chintapalli et al.[7] retrospectively evaluated CT scans from 27 patients suffering from diverticulitis and 31 with colon cancer. Five radiologists were blinded to the proven diagnosis. Pericolonic inflammation and segment involvement greater than 10

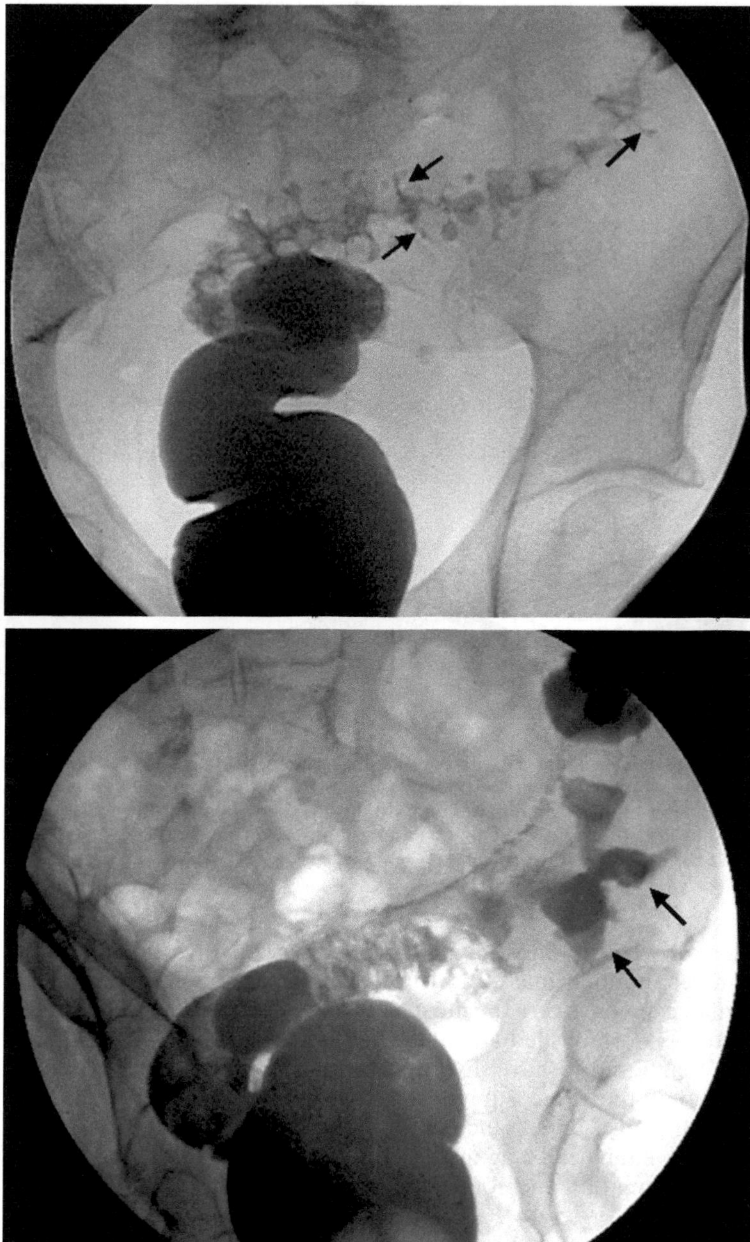

A

B

Figure 1 Contrast enema with water soluble contrast medium. **A**: Acute diverticulitis of the sigmoid colon; lumen stenosis, spasm, narrowing of diverticula orifice (→): length of involved segment > 10 cm. **B**: Diverticulitis of the sigmoid colon with contrast medium extravasation (→) indicating perforation

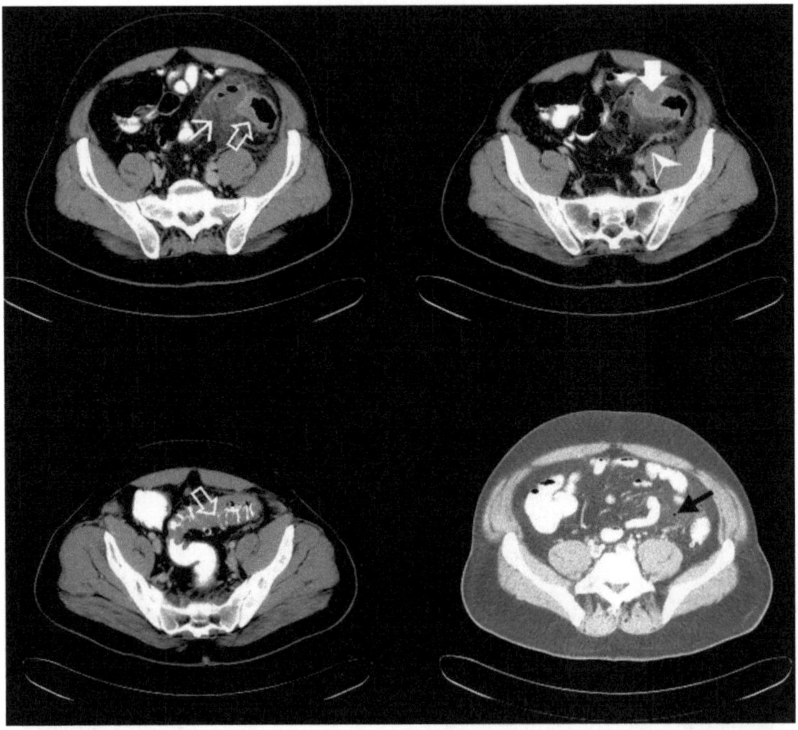

Figure 2 Acute diverticulitis, CT with contrast medium application rectally and intravenously. Length of the involved segment >10 cm. Typical signs with lumen stenosis and bowel wall thickening (open white arrow), fat stranding (thin white arrow), fascial thickening (arrowhead), abscess within the wall (solid white arrow) and small free air bubble (black arrow). Diagnosis, abscess and perforation verified by surgery

cm in length were the most significant findings for diverticulitis. Pericolonic lymph nodes, luminal mass and 'shoulder formation' – similar to the 'apple core' sign in enemas – were the most significant findings for colon cancer (Table 2). Five readers established a confidence category (Table 3): If the patient was definitely diagnosed to have diverticulitis or colon cancer, all diagnoses were correct, but if the three equivocal categories were included, there was an overlap with the CT appearance in 51%. Thus, for half of the group, CT could offer only an equivocal diagnosis and was not able to distinguish definitely between inflammation and colon cancer.

MAGNETIC RESONANCE TOMOGRAPHY

There are only a few reports available regarding MRI in diverticulosis or diverticulitis[8–10]. Schreyer et al.[8] examined 14 consecutive patients with clinical suspected diverticulitis. In all patients a water–gadolinium–DPTA

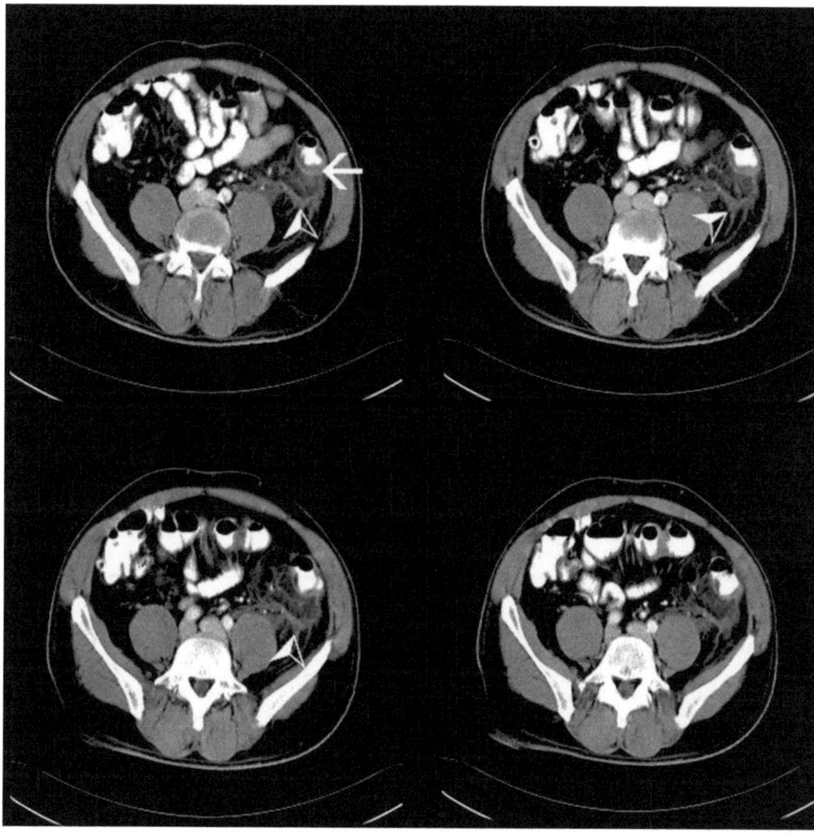

Figure 3 CT with contrast medium application rectally and intravenously. Clinical signs and laboratory results worrisome for acute diverticulitis. Excentric bowel wall thickening (arrow) of descending colon, worrisome for cancer. Extensive thickening of the lateroconal fascia (arrowhead) and fat stranding are more typical for diverticulitis, which was verified by surgery

mixture was administered rectally, and N-butyl-scopolamine was given intravenously to reduce bowel peristalsis. The criteria for diverticulitis were identical with those for CT (Figure 4). Patients with perforation, verified by CT, were excluded from this study because of the potential (and unknown) side-effects of gadolinium–DPTA in cases of unexpected perforation not seen on CT. In this preliminary study MRI colonography revealed the same diagnosis as CT in all six patients suffering from diverticulitis. In the study of Heverhagen et al.[9] the similar MRI technique was used in 20 patients with suspected diverticulitis, and MRI was diagnostic in all but one patient. Cobben et al.[10] described MRI imaging in five patients with right-sided diverticulitis, and recommended MRI imaging as a valuable alternative to CT in young or pregnant patients who have suspected appendicitis and an equivocal ultrasound result.

Table 1 Sensitivity and specifity of individual signs on helical CT

	No. of patients	*Sensitivity (%)*	*Specificity (%)*
Bowel wall thickening	109	96	91
Fat stranding	108	95	90
Diverticula	104	91	67
Fascial thickening	37	50	100
Free air	34	30	100
Free fluid	51	45	97
Inflamed diverticula	49	43	100

Retrospective analysis vs prospective interpretation in 114 patients.

From Kircher et al.[6]

Table 2 Diverticulitis vs colon cancer: differentiation with helical CT findings

	Diverticulitis 40 patients	*Colon cancer 32 patients*	*p-Values*
Length of segment			
<5 cm	2 (5%)	10 (2%)	>0.0025
5–10 cm	30 (75%)	21 (66%)	>0.0025
>10 cm	8 (20%)	1 (1%)	>0.0025
Pericolonic inflammation	38 (95%)	21 (60%)	<0.005
Pericolonic oedema	31 (78%)	11 (34%)	<0.003
Fluid in the root of mesentery	20 (50%)	3 (9%)	
Extraluminal fluid or air	12 (30%)	2 (6%)	<0.01
Excentric wall thickening	10 (25%)	16 (50%)	<0.0026
Shoulder formation	1 (3%)	16 (50%	>0.001
Lymph nodes	3 (8%)	23 (27%)	<0.001

Prospective evaluation. From Chintapalli et al.[7].

Table 3 Confidence category, five readers

CT diagnosis	*No. of patients*	*Diverticulitis*	*Cancer*
Definitely diverticulitis	16	16	–
Probably diverticulitis	18	16	2
Indeterminate	11	7	4
Probably malignant	1	5	–
Definitely malignant	21	–	21

From Chintapalli et al.[7].

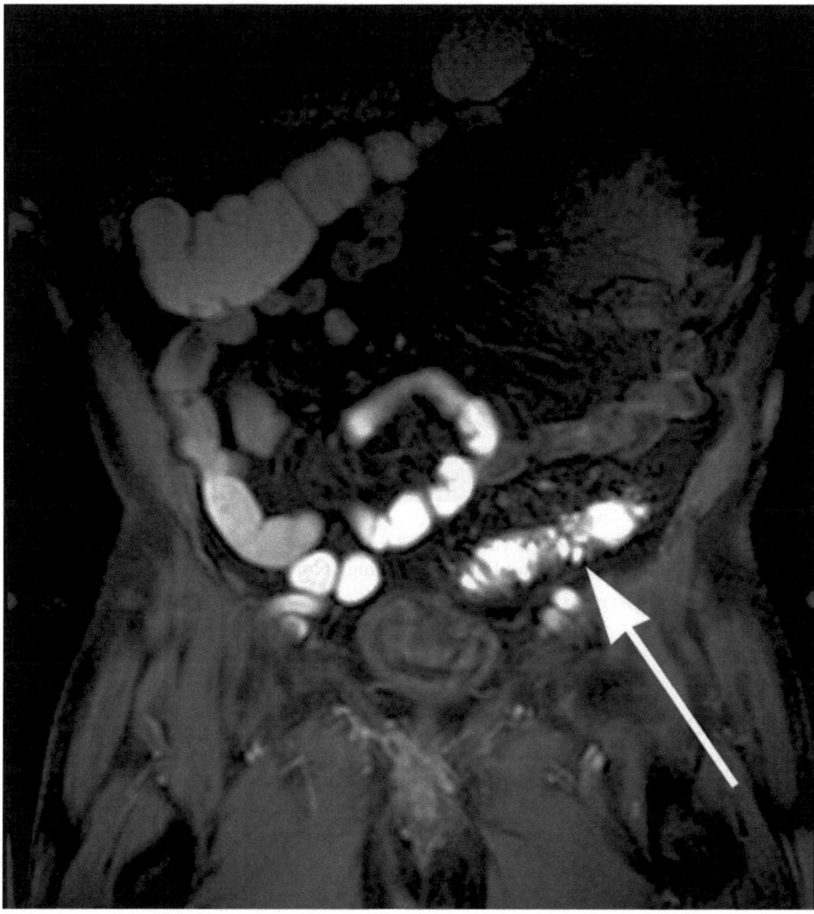

Figure 4 Acute diverticulitis of the sigmoid colon, MRI: after intravenous application of contrast media the fat saturated two-dimensional-flash sequence shows bowel wall enhancement (→). Diverticulitis also verified by CT

MRI has a few disadvantages: patients with major abdominal pain may not tolerate the examination time of 20 min, which is significantly longer compared to helical CT; MRI is more sensitive for motion artefacts, and monitoring of very ill patients is more difficult in the MRI suite compared to CT. Another problem is the identification of free abdominal air; there are no studies assessing free abdominal air with MRI; we therefore consider MRI as an alternative method to spiral CT in selected cases only. If patients should undergo elective surgery in the symptom-free interval, MRI has a potential to demonstrate all diverticula in the entire colon as well as contrast enema studies, especially when volume rendering three-dimensional models are created (Figure 5)[8].

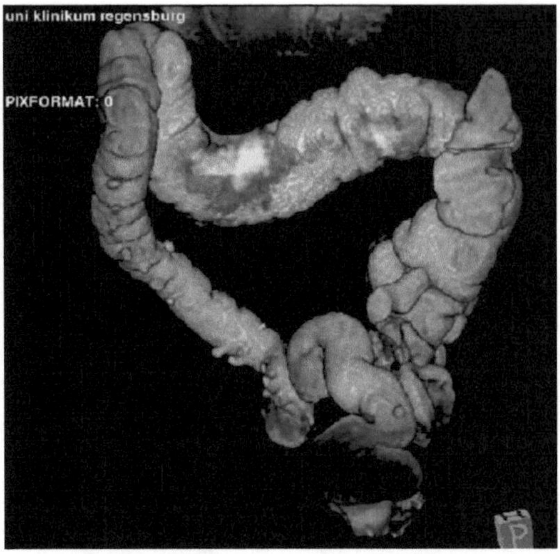

Figure 5 Diverticulosis, MRI. The volume-rendered three-dimensional model from a posterior view reveals diverticula of the sigmoid and descending colon

CONCLUSION

CT is a safe and cost-effective method with the additional potential to guide the drainage of abscesses. Moreover, it is an operator-independent technique with an excellent documentation. Thus, CT is the method of choice in many institutions. Ultrasound offers comparable results, is non-invasive and widely available, but operator-dependent, and the image quality is often insufficient in obese patients or in patients with meteorism. Both modalities, CT and ultrasound, are reliable methods to identify diverticulitis and their complications. MRI has a similar potential, but is more sensitive for motion artefacts; the sensitivity to identify free air bubbles is unknown. Further studies are necessary to define the role of MRI in the future.

References

1. Stollman NH, Raskin JB. Diagnosis and management of diverticular disease of the colon in adults. Am J Gastroenterol. 1999;94:3110–21.
2. Ahn SH, Mayo-Smith WW, Murphy BL, Reinert SE, Cronan J. Acute nontraumatic abdominal pain in adult patients: abdominal radiography compared with CT evaluation. Radiology. 2002;225:159–64.
3. Ambrosetti P, Jenny A, Becker C, Terrier TF, Morel P. Acute left colonic diverticulitis – compared performance of computed tomography and water-soluble contrast enema: prospective evaluation of 420 patients. Dis Colon Rectum. 2000;43:1363–7.
4. Stollmann N, Raskin JB. Diverticular disease of the colon. Lancet. 2004,363:631–9.

5. Pradel JA, Adell JF, Taourel P, Djafari M, Monnin-Delhom E, Bruel JM. Acute colonic diverticulitis: prospective comparative evaluation with US and CT. Radiology. 1997;205: 503.
6. Kircher MF, Rhea JT, Kihiczak D, Novelline RA. Frequency, sensitivity, and specificy of individual signs of diverticulitis on thin-section helical CT with colonic contrast material: experience with 312 cases. Am J Roentgenol. 2002;178:1313–18.
7. Chintapalli KN, Chopra S, Ghiatas AA, Esola CC, Fields SF, Dodd GD. Diverticulitis versus colon cancer: differentiation with helical CT findings. Radiology. 1999;210:429–35.
8. Schreyer AG, Fürst A, Agha A et al. Magnetic resonance imaging based colonography for diagnosis and assessment of diverticulosis and diverticulitis. Int J Colorectal Dis. 2004;19: 474–80.
9. Heverhaben JT, Zielke A, Ishaque N, Bohrer T, El-Sheik M, Klose KJ. Acute colonic diverticulitis: visualization in magnetic resonance imaging. Magn Reson Imaging. 2001;19: 1275–7.
10. Cobben LPJ, Groot I, Blickman JG, Puylaert JBCM. Right colonic diverticulitis: MR appearance. Abdom Imaging. 2003;28:794–8.

Section VI
Determinants of treatment

Chair: C.G.S. HÜSCHER and M. ZEITZ

13
Natural course of diverticular disease

M. Z. PANOS

EPIDEMIOLOGY

In Western industrialized populations diverticular disease of the colon (DD) is common, its prevalence ranging between 20% and 60%[1–3], in contrast to the populations of Asian countries where it is uncommon, ranging from 1% to 25%[4–6] and African countries where it is rare, ranging from 0% to 4%[7–9]. There is an increase in prevalence with age. DD is almost unknown in adolescents and its frequency rises from 2–29% in the under-40s, to 30–35% in those over 45 years and 42–66% in those over 85 years[1,2]. In addition, there is evidence, from comparisons of the results of studies performed in the first and second parts of the twentieth century, that the prevalence of the disease is increasing in Europe, Asia and Africa[10], and that the male to female ratio has changed from 3:1 to 1:1 over the same period[11,12]. Left-sided disease predominates in the West (90–95%),[13], whilst in Asian populations right-sided disease is more common (76%),[14]. As in the case of Western populations, the prevalence of DD in Asians increases with age and there is no gender difference[14]. A rising frequency of DD seems to parallel increasing industrialization and change to a Western diet and lifestyle. This is suggested by a series of Japanese studies which reported a rising prevalence of DD from 2.1% in 1967 to 5.4% in 1970, 23% in 1986 and 28% in 2000 (with right-sided colonic disease remaining predominant)[15,16], and is supported by the findings of a necropsy study of Japanese immigrants living in Hawaii in which diverticula were identified in 52% of specimens examined[17], in contrast to a finding of 1% as reported from a Japanese necropsy study of the same period[18]. There is also evidence from Africa that diverticular disease is increasing with urbanization, as suggested by a study from sub-Saharan Africa which reported a 4% prevalence in native Blacks and 21–31% in Whites[26]. This level of prevalence in African Blacks is higher than previously reported[7–9], even though it remains much lower than in Whites living in the same community. The last observation, along with the finding from the Asian studies in which right-sided colonic disease continues to predominate despite a sharp rise in prevalence in Westernized Asian communities[17,18], suggests that, in addition to the major contributing environmental factors, which seem to be diet and a Western lifestyle, there is a genetic component to the disease.

DIET AND LIFESTYLE

Painter and Burkitt proposed that decreasing intake of fibre in the form of whole grains, vegetables and fruits, and increasing consumption of refined flour, jams, sugar and meat products, was responsible for lower stool volumes, slower gut transit times, higher intraluminal pressures and consequent gut wall thickening and hypersegmentation, all of which predisposed to the formation of diverticulae[7,10,19]. Two prospective studies support the fibre hypothesis. A study from the Oxford area found DD in 12% of vegetarians with a mean daily intake of 42 g fibre, as compared to 33% in non-vegetarians with a daily fibre intake of 21g[20]. The USA Health Professionals Follow-up Study, in which nearly 50 000 men were followed for 4 years, found an inverse correlation between incidence of symptomatic diverticulosis and intake of insoluble fibre, with a relative risk of 0.63[21]. In the same study no correlation was found between symptomatic DD and smoking, caffeine or alcohol consumption[22]. A case–control study from Greece, in addition to finding an association between low fibre intake and DD, reported an association between the consumption of meat and milk products and higher socioeconomic status and increased frequency of DD[23].

NATURAL HISTORY OF DD

Although the prevalence of DD increases with age, there does not seem to be a progression of the extent of colon affected, or an increase in the proportion of individuals with symptomatic disease with increasing age[24]. Patients with uncomplicated DD as an incidental finding appear to be no more likely (20–30%) to complain of non-specific abdominal symptoms (abdominal pain relieved by defaecation, altered stool frequency or consistency, or abdominal distension), than individuals without diverticuli[25]. Even though considerable overlap of symptoms with the irritable bowel syndrome (IBS), another common condition, may present difficulties in diagnosis and management, the natural history of patients with IBS-type symptoms appears to be independent of the presence or absence of diverticula[27].

Despite difficulties in discerning symptoms of DD from IBS, it seems that fibre supplementation in patients with symptomatic DD may be of benefit. In a prospective double-blind controlled trial of 18 patients with symptomatic DD, fibre supplementation resulted in significant symptom improvement over a 3-month follow-up period[28,29]. Findings from retrospective studies support a beneficial role for added fibre in symptomatic DD. A retrospective study by Leahy et al. of 72 patients admitted with symptoms DD, found that fibre supplementation resulted in a reduction in the incidence of complications and requirement for surgery[30]. In another retrospective study of 100 consecutive patients with complicated DD, Hyland and Taylor reported that 91% remained symptom-free on a high-fibre diet at a mean follow-up time of 6 years[31].

PROGNOSIS AND COMPLICATIONS

Perforation and abscess formation

In the majority of individuals with colonic diverticulae the disease is silent, with 70–80% remaining asymptomatic[2,14,19]. About 15–20% will develop diverticulitis or its complications[6,32]. Uncomplicated diverticulitis (peridiverticular inflammation without perforation) accounts for 75% of these cases whilst the remaining 25% comprises complications such as diverticular abscesses, perforation with peritonitis, fistulas and strictures[32]. These complications are almost invariably treated surgically[33]. Up to 41% of all patients with diverticulitis ultimately come to surgery[33]. On a first admission with acute diverticulitis, 65–85% will respond to medical treatment, the remainder requiring surgery with an overall mortality for a first admission of 1.3–5.7%. Those requiring surgery have a mortality of 12–17%[1,33,34]. Perforated diverticulitis (abscess or peritonitis) has an incidence 4/100 000 population per annum in the UK with a mortality rate of 28%, which is partly due to the high frequency of co-morbidity in an elderly population[35]. It is worth noting that of those presenting with diverticular perforation only 22% give a history of previous diverticular disease[35]. Risk factors identified as contributing to perforation of colonic diverticula include use of NSAID (RR 3.71)[35], immunosuppression as a result of either underlying disease (such as diabetes, renal failure, haematological malignancy, bone marrow suppression or infiltration, HIV disease), or drug-induced immunosuppression by chemotherapy, steroid treatment or immunosuppression post-transplant[36]. In one study, free perforation occurred in 43% of immuno-compromised patients with DD, as compared to a perforation rate of 14% in the immunocompetent control group, with a corresponding mortality rate of 39% and 2% respectively[37]. Obese, young, male patients with DD also have an increased risk of presenting with acute diverticulitis and perforation.

Most patients with diverticulitis present with a short duration of symptoms and only 8% give a history of previous attacks. In those who avoid surgery on the first admission the risk of recurrence is about 2% per year[33]. In the long term, one-third of patients will remain asymptomatic, one-third will have abdominal pain and one-third will have a further attack of diverticulitis or its complications[1,32]. Patients who recover from a second attack of diverticulitis without surgery have a 90% chance of a further attack[1]. On this evidence it seems reasonable to offer surgery to patients following a second attack of diverticulitis. Following sigmoid resection it is estimated that 3–15% of patients will develop recurrent symptoms, but only a minority require further surgery[38].

Diverticular haemorrhage

Diverticular haemorrhage (DH) occurs in 5–15% of those with DD and accounts for 40% of all cases of lower gastrointestinal haemorrhage[32,39]. The risk of bleeding increases with age and use of NSAID (RR 2.24) and paracetamol (RR 1.81)[40]. In one-third of cases the bleeding is massive and 7% require surgery, with a mortality rate of 2.2%. The majority of diverticular haemorrhages are self-limiting but up to 40% will continue to bleed or rebleed during the index admission[41]. In cases where surgery is avoided during the first episode of DH, the risk of recurrence at 4 years is 25%. After two episodes of DH the risk of rebleeding rises to 50%[41]. There is evidence to suggest that in Western populations, the risk of DH is higher in those with right-sided colonic disease[42] (even though in this group left-sided disease predominates (90–95%)). In Asian populations, where right-sided disease predominates (76%), right-sided bleeding accounts for 40–50% of cases of DH[43].

Diverticular fistulas

The reported incidence of internal fistulas in patients with a history of diverticulitis is 2%. A fistula arises if a diverticular phlegmon or abscess ruptures into an adjacent organ. Colovesical fistulas account for 65% and colovaginal for 25%. Involvement of other organs (coloenteric, colocolonic, colosalpingeal colocholecystic and colocutaneous) accounts for the remaining 10%[44]. In the differential diagnosis other causes of fistulating disease, such as Crohn's disease, malignancy, radiation damage and ischaemic colitis, should be considered[44]. In fit patients the treatment of choice is surgical.

Obstruction

Small bowel obstruction in acute diverticulitis is usually due to involvement of one or more loops in the inflammatory mass or paralytic ileus due to peritoneal irritation. It usually resolves with successful medical management of the diverticulitis. Large bowel obstruction accounts for only up to 30% of all large bowel obstructions and is a result of oedema, colonic spasm and inflammation; it is especially likely in chronic disease with the resultant fibrosis and narrowed lumen[44]. Medical management is usually enough to resolve the obstruction and surgical intervention is necessary only in cases of complete obstruction. Other causes of bowel obstruction such as malignancy need to be excluded[44].

Diverticular stricture

Recurrent attacks of diverticulitis may result in fibrosis and strictures. Onset of symptoms is insidious, often with change in bowel habit and abdominal bloating. Other causes of stricture need to be considered, such as bowel malignancy, extrinsic compression by urological or gynaecological malignancy, Crohn's disease, radiotherapy or ischaemia[44].

CONCLUSIONS

Diverticular disease is common in industrialized countries and is mostly asymptomatic. Complications occur in about 20% of patients and of those only 25–35% overall suffer complications or recurring attacks. Understanding the natural history of the disease will enable appropriate interventions in order to prevent recurrent attacks and complications.

References

1. Parks TG. Natural history of diverticular disease of the colon. Clin Gastroenterol. 1975;4:53–69.
2. Manousos ON et al. Prevalence of diverticulosis in the general population of the Oxford area. Br Med J. 1967;3;762–3.
3. Eastwood MA et al. Variation in the incidence of diverticular disease in the city of Edinburgh. Gut. 1977;18:571–4.
4. Vajrabukka et al. Diverticular disease of the colon in a Far Eastern community. Dis Colon Rectum. 1980;23:151–4.
5. Guo-Zong P et al. Diverticular disease of the colon in China. Chin Med J. 1984;97:391–4.
6. Kubo A et al. Clinical studies on diverticular disease of the colon. Jpn J Med. 1983;22:185–9.
7. Painter NS, Burkitt DP. Diverticular disease of the colon: a 20th century problem. Gastroenterology. 1975;1:3–21.
8. Archampong EQ et al. Diverticular disease in an indigenous African community. Ann R Coll Surg Engl. 1978;60:464–70.
9. Calder JF. Diverticular disease of the colon in Africans. Br Med J. 1979;1:1465–6.
10. Painter NS, Burkitt DP. Diverticular disease of the colon: a deficiency disease of Western civilisation. Br Med J. 1971;2:450–4.
11. Chalmers K et al. Diverticular disease of the colon in Scottish hospitals over a decade. Health Bull. 1983;40:32–41.
12. Kyle J, Davidson AI. The changing pattern of hospital admissions for diverticular disease of the colon. Br J Surg. 1975;62:537–41.
13. Hughes LE. Postmortem study of diverticular disease of the colon. Gut. 1969;10:336–51.
14. Narasaka T et al. Statistical analysis of diverticulosis of the colon. Tohuku J Exp Med. 1975;115:271–5.
15. Nakada I et al. Diverticular disease of the colon at a regional general hospital in Japan. Dis Colon Rectum. 1995;38:755–9.
16. Miura S et al. Recent trends in diverticulosis of the right colon in Japan. Dis Col Rectum. 2000;43:1383–9.
17. Stemmerman GN, Yatani R. Diverticulosis and polyps of the large intestine. A necropsy study of Hawaii Japanese. Cancer. 1973;31:1260–70.
18. Sato E et al. Polyps and diverticulosis of the large bowel in autopsy population of Akita prefecture with Miyaki. Cancer. 1976;37:1316–21.
19. Burkitt DP et al. Effect of dietary fibre on stools and transit times and its role in the causation of disease. Lancet. 1979;2:1408–11.
20. Gear JS et al. Symptomless diverticular disease and intake of dietary fibre. Lancet. 1979; I:511–14.
21. Aldoori WH et al. A prospective study of dietary fibre types and symptomatic diverticular disease in men. J Nutr. 1998;128:714–19.
22. Aldoori WH et al. A prospective study of alcohol smoking caffeine and the risk of symptomatic diverticular disease in men. Ann Epidemiol. 1995;5:221–8.
23. Manousos O et al. Diet and other factors in the aetiology of diverticulosis: an epidemiological study in Greece. Gut. 1985;26:544–9.
24. Horner JL. Natural history of diverticulosis of the colon. Am J Dig Dis. 1958;5:343–6.
25. Thompson WG et al. Does uncomplicated diverticular disease produce symptoms? Dig Dis Sci. 1982;27:605–8.
26. Walker ARP, Segal I. Effects of transition on bowel diseases in sub-Saharan Africans. Eur J Gastroenterol Hepatol. 1997;9:207–10.
27. Otte JJ et al. Irritable bowel syndrome and symptomatic diverticular disease- different diseases? Am J Gastroenterol. 1986;81:529–31.
28. Brodribb AJM, Humphreys DM. Diverticular disease: three studies. Part II. Treatment with bran. Br Med J. 1976;1:425–8.
29. Brodribb AJM. Treatment of symptomatic diverticular disease with a high fibre diet. Lancet. 1977;I:664–6.
30. Leahy AL et al. High fibre diet in symptomatic diverticular disease of the colon. Ann R Coll Surg Engl. 1985;67:173–4.

31. Hyland JMP, Taylor I. Does high fibre diet prevent the complications of diverticular disease? Br J Surg. 1980;67:77–9.
32. Young-Fadok TM et al. Colonic diverticular disease. Curr Probl Surg. 2000;37:457–514.
33. Sarin S, Boulos PB. Long term outcome of patients presenting with acute complications of diverticular disease. Ann R Coll Surg Engl. 1994;76:117–20.
34. Elliott TB et al. Five year audit of acute complications of diverticular disease. Br J Surg. 1997;84:535–9.
35. Hart AR et al. How frequently do large bowel diverticula perforate? Eur J Gastroenterol Hepatol. 2000;12:661–5.
36. Perkins JD et al. Comparison of treatment in immunocompromised and non-immunocompromised patients. Am J Surg. 1984;148:745–8.
37. Tyau ES et al. Acute diverticulitis: acomplicated problem in the immunocompromised patient. Arch Surg. 1991;126:855–9.
38. Farmakis N et al. The 5-year natural history of complicated diverticular disease. Br J Surg. 1994;81:733–5.
39. Almy DP, Howell DA. Diverticular disease of the colon N Engl J Med. 1980;302:324–31.
40. Aldoori WH et al. Use of acetaminofen and non-steroidal anti-inflammatory drugs: a prospective study and the risk of of symptomatic diverticular disease in men. Arch Fam Med. 1998;7:255–60.
41. McGuire HH. Bleeding colonic diverticula:a reappraisal of natural history and management. Ann Surg. 1994;220:653–6.
42. Stollman NH, Raskin JB. Diagnosis and management of diverticular disease in adults. Ad Hoc Practice Prameters Committee for the American College of Gastroenterology. Am J Gastroenterol. 1999;94:3110–21.
43. So JB et al. Right sided colonic diverticular disease as a source of lower g.i. bleeding. Am Surg. 1999;65:299–302.
44. Fearnhead NS, Mortensen N. Clinical features and differential diagnosis of diverticular disease. Best Pract Res Clin Gastroenterol. 2002;16:4:577–93.

14
Pain in diverticular diseases

R. C. SPILLER

INCIDENCE OF PAIN IN DIVERTICULOSIS

While diverticulosis is extremely common in the Western world, affecting 35% of those over the age of 50 in the United Kingdom[1] and 50–66% of patients over age 80[2], the majority of these patients do not suffer pain. The precise proportion of patients suffering from pain is not clear from the literature, but in one very large prospective study of a cohort of 47 888 US health professionals during a 4-year follow-up, 385 subjects developed new symptomatic diverticular disease, an incidence of 1.8 per 1000 patient years.

While prospective studies are undoubtedly the best way to obtain the true incidence, these are rarely possible. In our own approach to answer this question we examined all the barium enemas performed at University Hospital over a 4-month period and identified 411 with diverticulosis. After excluding those who died or had cancer, we sent a postal bowel symptom questionnaire to 378 individuals, of whom 261 replied (response rate 69%). This was, as expected, a largely elderly population, age 69 (36–91) (median, range) with a slight female predominance, 144 females and 117 males. The proportion reporting recurrent abdominal pain varied according to the indication for the enema. In those in whom the enema was performed for reasons unrelated to abdominal pain – such as cancer screening, anaemia or rectal bleeding – the incidence was around 15%, while in those in whom a change in bowel habit was a reason for the enema the incidence of pain was 35%. If only 15% are symptomatic this suggests that diverticulosis *per se* does not cause symptoms, but requires some other factor(s). This idea fits with clinical experience in which the number or extent of diverticula appears to bear no relation to the severity of symptoms. It also fits with the finding that most right-sided diverticula present with bleeding rather than pain[3,4], and that the incidence of abdominal pain in those found to have diverticular generally does not differ from the normal population[5], particularly in areas where right-sided colonic diverticula are common[6].

PATTERNS OF ABDOMINAL PAIN IN DIVERTICULOSIS

We distinguished two sorts of abdominal pain in our survey[7]. One was a recurrent but short-lived pain similar to that experienced by patients with irritable bowel syndrome, and the second was a more prolonged pain characterized by: (1) duration >24 h; (2) interference with normal activities; and (3) usually a medical consultation. Ninety-four of our patients described recurrent short-lived pain which occurred with a frequency (median, interquartile range) of 5 (2–13) days per month. The median duration was 3 (0.1–12) h. This was quite different from the prolonged pain, which had a median duration of 3 (2–5) days. During these episodes of pain, 33 out of 51 patients sought medical attention and 25 out of 50 consultations led to the prescription of antibiotics, suggesting that the medical practitioner suspected acute diverticulitis. We examined associated bowel features in the 94 patients with recurrent short-lived pain and found that both loose and hard stools were common, as were straining and urgency, sometimes in the same patient (see Table 1).

Table 1 Bowel symptoms in 94 patients with painful diverticulosis (adapted from ref. 7)

Symptoms	*N (%)*	*Frequency in days/week; median (range)*
Loose stool	50 (53.2)	5(1-7)
Hard stool	50 (53.2)	2(1-7)
Straining	41 (43.6)	3(1-7)
Urgency	45 (47.9)	3(1-7)
Incontinence	16 (17.0)	3(1-7)
Mucus per rectum	20 (21.3)	2(1-7)
Bloating	55 (58.5)	3(1-7)

RISK FACTORS FOR PREDICTING THE DEVELOPMENT OF RECURRENT ABDOMINAL PAIN

Neither age nor gender, nor the severity of radiological appearance, predicted the occurrence of pain or abnormalities of bowel habit. The only predictor of recurrent pain was a past history of prolonged pain, which we took to represent acute diverticulitis. Of those 51 with such a history, 31 (61%) had recurrent pain, while of the 210 without such a history, only 63 (30%) had pain, giving a relative risk of 2.0. The results of this study then led us to perform a further prospective study of 26 patients admitted with acute diverticulitis documented by fever, increased white cell count and abdominal tenderness with guarding. Over the next 2-year period 18 out of the 26 patients experienced new recurrent short-lived pain[7].

MECHANISM OF PAIN IN DIVERTICULOSIS

The bowel is relatively insensitive to most stimuli, and patients rarely report symptoms during cautery or biopsy of the bowel mucosa. Unlike somatic tissue, burning and cutting is not readily perceived; however, stretching is a potent and painful stimulus. Studies performed in the stomach[8] with muscle relaxants indicate that it is an increase in wall tension induced by distension which causes symptoms, though during colorectal distension with a balloon, mechanical deformation appears more important than wall tension[9]. Wall tension may also increase because of high-amplitude pressure contractions (HAPC). Studies in irritable bowel syndrome have indicated that these HAPC are often associated with pain, though interestingly similar amplitude contractions in normal individuals are not perceived[10]. Plainly, then, increased wall tension or deformation is not sufficient to induce a sensation of pain, which also requires visceral hypersensitivity. One factor which can lead to sensitization is inflammation. Under these circumstances animal studies have indicated that both the threshold and the response to colorectal distension are enhanced (for review see ref.11), so that pain is now induced by normal pressure contractions. One of the most reliable stimuli for colonic contractions is eating[12], which may explain why patients with diverticular disease often report crampy left iliac fossa pain soon after meals.

POSTPRANDIAL COLONIC RESPONSE IN DIVERTICULAR DISEASE

An extensive study on 115 patients with colonic diverticular disease examined the association between symptoms and postprandial contractions. A manometry probe was placed in the left colon and the motility index recorded both basally and after a meal[13]. The patients were divided into 30 asymptomatic with diverticulosis and 30 with symptomatic but uncomplicated diverticulosis (SUDD) and 55 with symptomatic complicated diverticular disease (SCDD). When compared with 30 healthy controls, basal values were elevated in the SUDD and SCDD patients but much more markedly elevated in the postprandial period in both SUDD and SCDD (Figure 1). This particular study did not document whether the subjects experienced pain at the time of the study, so the study by Bassotti et al.[14] is of particular value. These workers studied 12 patients with symptomatic but uncomplicated diverticular disease and compared them with 20 healthy controls. They performed 24-h ambulatory left colonic manometry, which is necessary to capture infrequent bouts of pain. They found that the diverticular patients had an increased proportion of their total activity recorded as a regular two to three contractions per min. This increase was particularly marked in the sigmoid colon where 63% of the activity was regular two or three cycles per minute compared with 49% in controls. Interestingly, the amplitude of contractions was similar: controls 25 ± 9 mmHg and diverticular patients 29 ± 11 mmHg. They then performed a calculation of symptom-associated probability. Each individual record was divided into 5-min epochs and the presence of pain and/or regular contractions recorded in each epoch. The Fisher exact test was used to calculate the probability p of the

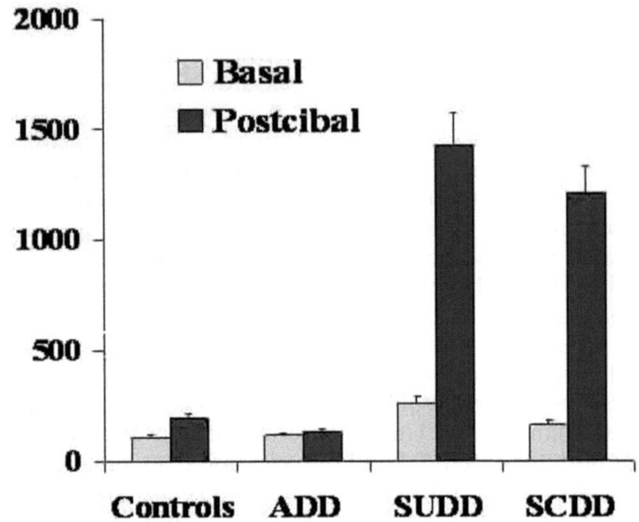

Figure 1 Motility index 3 h before and 3 h after a standard 1000 kcal test meal in 30 healthy controls, 30 asymptomatic (ADD), 30 symptomatic uncomplicated (SUDD) and 55 symptomatic complicated (SCDD) diverticular disease patients. Redrawn from Cortesini et al.[13]

association occurring by chance. The symptom-associated probability is $1 - p \times 100$. Four of the patients and none of the controls experienced pain during the study. The symptom-associated probability in the patients was 97–99%, suggesting that contractions were very closely associated with the presence of pain. However, since the amplitude to contractions was the same in patients and controls, this provides further evidence for visceral hypersensitivity in symptomatic diverticular disease. Visceral hypersensitivity is often assessed by gauging the pressure required to induce pain during rectal distension with a balloon. Clemens and colleagues[15] used this technique to study 10 asymptomatic and 11 symptomatic uncomplicated diverticular disease. Visceral sensitivity was assessed in both the rectum and the sigmoid colon. Interestingly, in both regions the perception score was higher at any given pressure for the symptomatic diverticular patients compared with both the asymptomatic diverticular patients and healthy controls. This difference was slightly exaggerated in the sigmoid colon after meals, which are often followed by symptoms in patients with diverticular disease.

INFLAMMATION AND VISCERAL HYPERSENSITIVITY

There is now a very large amount of literature indicating clearly that inflammation leads to visceral hypersensitivity in laboratory animals. The models have varied pathology but show a similar effect. The most widely used model, *Trichinella spiralis*, produces an acute inflammation as the worm burrows through the jejunal mucosa. The worm has left the gut by about 14 days and the inflammation has largely subsided by 28 days. Several groups have demonstrated persistent abnormal motility with features somewhat reminiscent of diverticular disease including muscular hypertrophy[16], uncoordinated contractions and visceral hypersensitivity[17]. There is evidence of up-regulation of tachykinins, particularly substance P[16,18] and evidence of impaired release of neurotransmitters including norepinephrine and acetylcholine[19,20]. This appears to be mediated by cytokines, particularly interleukin 1[19–21]. There is an associated hypersensitivity to distension[17], and in our own recent studies there is also evidence of increased afferent nerve firing in response to intestinal distension mediated by serotonin release[22]. Whilst this model, which is largely T cell-driven, has been useful to define mechanisms, it is somewhat different from the more acute diverticular-associated inflammation. This is perhaps better modelled by the colitis induced by rectal installation of trinitrobenzene sulphonic acid (TNBS) or the ingestion of dextran sodium sulphate (DSS), which both induce damage to the mucosa followed by an inflammatory response to luminal bacteria, which then gradually subsides over a period of 3–4 weeks. This too is associated with muscle thickening, abnormal motility, impaired neurotransmitter release[23,24] and evidence of nerve damage[25]. Serotonin availability is increased[23] and, after initial decline, substance P increases[25].

OTHER CAUSES OF VISCERAL HYPERSENSITIVITY

The widespread recognition that patients suffering from irritable bowel syndrome (IBS) have increased incidence of psychological distress has led many to suggest that visceral hypersensitivity may be largely centrally determined[26]. Animal models of anxiety and stress (maternal separation and water avoidance) clearly show that these factors induce hyper-responsiveness to colorectal distension[11]. Human studies have also shown altered central processing of visceral stimuli, possibly reflecting a conditioned fear of such stimuli (reviewed in ref. 26). No data exist as to the effect of anxiety and depression on symptoms in diverticular disease, but it is probably as important as in IBS, particularly in this age group which is frequently exposed to bereavement and health-related anxiety.

ROLE OF NITRIC OXIDE IN INFLAMMATION-ASSOCIATED DYSMOTILITY

Using the TNBS colitis model, Depoortere et al.[27] showed a decrease in neuronal nitric oxide synthetase expression (nNOS) and a loss of nitrergic and adrenergic neurotransmission with profound alterations in response to serotonin, switching from a general inhibitory response to an excitatory one[27]. In the DSS colitis model in rats, Mizuta et al.[28] also showed a marked impairment in non-adrenergic/non-cholinergic (NANC) relaxation associated with a decrease in nNOS and a selective loss of nitrergic neurons.

ROLE OF NITRIC OXIDE IN DYSMOTILITY IN DIVERTICULAR DISEASE

Tomita et al.[29] examined 11 sigmoid colons with diverticulosis which had been resected for either cancer or symptomatic diverticular disease. Unfortunately, these different sources are not distinguished. Muscle contractions of excised muscle strips were recorded in an organ bath in response to electrical stimulation. They showed that, compared with controls, diverticular patients were half as likely to respond to electrical field stimulation with relaxation, a response normally mediated through nitrergic neurons. This difference remained under NANC conditions and no relaxations were seen in any of the preparations when treated with tetrodotoxin toxin, indicating that all the responses were mediated via neuronal activation. In order to demonstrate the importance of nitric oxide they then examined the dose–response to L-arginine, a precursor of nitric oxide. Increasing doses of L-arginine increased the proportion of samples showing relaxation on electrical field stimulation, but this was persistently less in diverticular patients compared with controls. Similarly when a nitric oxide synthetase blocker L-NG-nitroarginine (L-NNA) was given at increasing doses, the proportion showing relaxation fell, again with diverticular patients showing much less relation at all concentrations. This might well be important in the disorders of defecation seen in diverticular disease, because relaxation of the sigmoid colon may well be important in allowing the passage of stool from sigmoid colon to the rectum. Several studies have indicated high pressures in this region in patients with symptomatic diverticular disease[30] and resecting this region may be associated with marked diarrhoea[31], suggesting that the sigmoid region is acting as a brake on normal transit.

EVIDENCE OF ALTERED CHOLINERGIC AND SUBSTANCE P SENSITIVITY AS A CAUSE OF DYSMOTILITY IN DIVERTICULOSIS

Regrettably, the data in this area are quite conflicting, and what is available is based on very small numbers. Golder and colleagues[32] examined specimens from 10 patients who had incidental diverticular disease at the time of resection for cancer. These were therefore not symptomatic diverticular patients. They showed increased muscarinic type 3 receptor (M3) staining, together with a decrease in area staining for the marker of cholinergic neurons, choline-acetyltransferase (ChAT) when expressed as a percentage of the pan-neuronal marker PGP9.5; this was 17% in patients with diverticular disease compared with 47% in controls. The sensitivity to acetylcholine was increased in the patients, which led these authors to suggest that cholinergic denervation might be a feature of these patients. Whether this is cause or effect is uncertain; Liu and colleagues[33] examined the substance P receptor in circular muscle from diverticular-bearing colons. Contractile responses to substance P were considerably reduced in the diverticular disease[31]. The problem with these studies is that in no case were the subject's symptoms recorded, and it may well be that the pharmacology and innervation of patients with uncomplicated diverticulosis is quite different from that of symptomatic diverticulosis, particularly when it has been preceded by an episode of acute inflammation.

CHANGES IN MUCOSAL NEUROPEPTIDES IN SYMPTOMATIC AND ASYMPTOMATIC DIVERTICULOSIS PATIENTS

In our studies we examined changes in mucosal neuropeptides in 17 symptomatic and 15 asymptomatic diverticulosis patients. Our previous work has demonstrated similarities in the expression of the tachykinins in both the mucosa and the myenteric plexus using archival resected material. We found that there were increases in substance P staining and in galanin in the mucosa of symptomatic individuals[34]. Mucosal histology was normal and there was no evidence of ongoing inflammation. This therefore suggests that in symptomatic patients there has been some alteration in neuropeptide expression, possibly secondary to inflammation. Galanin is expressed in injured nerves and may merely be a marker of previous nerve damage, though recent studies suggest it also has a role in controlling intestinal secretions[35] and visceral sensation.

IMPLICATIONS FOR FUTURE RESEARCH AND TREATMENT

If pain and visceral hypersensitivity in diverticular patients are due to altered innervation and neuropeptide expression then treatments should be directed at this abnormality. Tachykinin antagonists, particularly neurokinin-2 receptor antagonists, have been shown in rodents to inhibit increased afferent firing[36] and reduce behavioural responses[37] in inflammatory hypersensitivity, so it would be reasonable to try these in humans. Other approaches would include a more vigorous attempt to inhibit ongoing inflammation at the time of acute inflammation. Anti-inflammatory drugs such as mesalazine should also be considered, as uncontrolled pilot data look promising[38]. Certainly these approaches need randomized, placebo-controlled studies, and offer the opportunity for exciting new developments.

SUMMARY

1. Diverticulosis alone does not cause pain.

2. It is important to distinguish episodic prolonged pain due to acute diverticular inflammation from the much more frequent, recurrent, but short-lived non-inflammatory pain.

3. Symptomatic patients with diverticulosis show increased postprandial motility and a hypersensitivity to colorectal distensions.

4. Episodes of acute diverticulosis increase the risk of recurrent short-lived pain.

5. Symptomatic patients show abnormal expression and responses to neuropeptides.

6. Visceral hypersensitivity and abnormal innervation could be a new target for therapy in this poorly understood condition.

References

1. Manousos ON, Truelove SC, Lumsden K. Prevalence of colonic diverticulosis in general population of Oxford area. Br Med J. 1967;3:762–3.
2. Stollman NH, Raskin JB. Diagnosis and management of diverticular disease of the colon in adults. Ad Hoc Practice Parameters Committee of the American College of Gastroenterology. Am J Gastroenterol. 1999;94:3110–21.
3. Ryan P. Changing concepts in diverticular disease. Dis Colon Rectum. 1983;26:12–18.
4. Wong SK, Ho YH, Leong AP et al. Clinical behavior of complicated right-sided and left-sided diverticulosis. Dis Colon Rectum. 1997;40:344–8.
5. Thompson WG, Patel DG, Tao H et al. Does uncomplicated diverticular disease produce symptoms? Dig Dis Sci. 1982;27:605–8.
6. Chan CC, Lo KK, Chung EC et al. Colonic diverticulosis in Hong Kong: distribution pattern and clinical significance. Clin Radiol. 1998;53:842–4.
7. Simpson J, Neal KR, Scholefield JH et al. Patterns of pain in diverticular disease and the influence of acute diverticulitis. Eur J Gastroenterol Hepatol. 2003;15:1005–10.
8. Distrutti E, Azpiroz F, Soldevilla A et al. Gastric wall tension determines perception of gastric distention. Gastroenterology. 1999;116:1035–42.
9. Drewes AM, Petersen P, Rossel P et al. Sensitivity and distensibility of the rectum and sigmoid colon in patients with irritable bowel syndrome. Scand J Gastroenterol. 2001;36: 827–32.
10. Chey WY, Jin HO, Lee MH et al. Colonic motility abnormality in patients with irritable bowel syndrome exhibiting abdominal pain and diarrhea. Am J Gastroenterol. 2001;96: 1499–506.
11. Mayer EA, Collins SM. Evolving pathophysiologic models of functional gastrointestinal disorders. Gastroenterology. 2002;122:2032–48.
12. Rao SS, Kavelock R, Beaty J et al. Effects of fat and carbohydrate meals on colonic motor response. Gut. 2000;46:205–11.
13. Cortesini C, Pantalone D. Usefulness of colonic motility study in identifying patients at risk for complicated diverticular disease. Dis Colon Rectum. 1991;34:339–42.
14. Bassotti G, Battaglia E, De Roberto G et al. Alterations in colonic motility and relationship to pain in colonic diverticulosis. Clin Gastroenterol Hepatol. 2005;3:248–53.

15. Clemens CH, Samsom M, Roelofs J et al. Colorectal visceral perception in diverticular disease. Gut. 2004;53:717–22.
16. Vermillion DL, Collins SM. Increased responsiveness of jejunal longitudinal muscle in *Trichinella*-infected rats. Am J Physiol. 1988;254:G124–9.
17. Bercik P, Wang L, Verdu EF et al. Visceral hyperalgesia and intestinal dysmotility in a mouse model of postinfective gut dysfunction. Gastroenterology. 2004;127:179–87.
18. Swain MG, Agro A, Blennerhassett P et al. Increased levels of substance P in the myenteric plexus of *Trichinella*-infected rats. Gastroenterology. 1992;102:1913–19.
19. Collins SM, Blennerhassett P, Vermillion DL et al. Impaired acetylcholine release in the inflamed rat intestine is T cell independent. Am J Physiol. 1992;263:G198–201.
20. Swain MG, Blennerhassett PA, Collins SM. Impaired sympathetic nerve function in the inflamed rat intestine. Gastroenterology. 1991;100:675–82.
21. Hurst S, Collins SM. Interleukin-1 beta modulation of norepinephrine release from rat myenteric nerves. Am J Physiol. 1993;264:G30–5.
22. Keating C, Foley S, Rieff-Marginiec A et al. Time dependent changes in jejunal afferent mechanosensitivity in mice infected with the nematode *Trichinella spiralis*. Gastroenterology. 2005;125(Suppl. 2):A10 (Abstract).
23. O'Hara JR, Ho W, Linden DR et al. Enteroendocrine cells and 5-HT availability are altered in mucosa of guinea pigs with TNBS ileitis. Am J Physiol Gastrointest Liver Physiol. 2004; 287:G998–1007.
24. Jacobson K, McHugh K, Collins SM. The mechanism of altered neural function in a rat model of acute colitis. Gastroenterology. 1997;112:156–62.
25. Miampamba M, Sharkey KA. Distribution of calcitonin gene-related peptide, somatostatin, substance P and vasoactive intestinal polypeptide in experimental colitis in rats. Neurogastroenterol Motil. 1998;10:315–29.
26. Whitehead WE, Palsson OS. Is rectal pain sensitivity a biological marker for irritable bowel syndrome? Psychological influences on pain perception. Gastroenterology. 1998;115:1263–71.
27. Depoortere I, Thijs T, Peeters TL. Generalized loss of inhibitory innervation reverses serotonergic inhibition into excitation in a rabbit model of TNBS-colitis. Br J Pharmacol. 2002;135:2011–19.
28. Mizuta Y, Isomoto H, Takahashi T. Impaired nitrergic innervation in rat colitis induced by dextran sulfate sodium. Gastroenterology. 2000;118:714–23.
29. Tomita R, Fujisaki S, Tanjoh K et al. Role of nitric oxide in the left-sided colon of patients with diverticular disease. Hepatogastroenterology. 2000;47:692–6.
30. Trotman IF, Misiewicz JJ. Sigmoid motility in diverticular disease and the irritable bowel syndrome. Gut. 1988;29:218–22.
31. Bassotti G, De Roberto G, Chistolini F et al. Case report: Colonic manometry reveals abnormal propulsive behaviour after anterior resection of the rectum. Dig Liver Dis. 2005; 37:124–8.
32. Golder M, Burleigh DE, Belai A et al. Smooth muscle cholinergic denervation hypersensitivity in diverticular disease. Lancet. 2003;361:1945–51.
33. Liu L, Shang F, Markus I et al. Roles of substance P receptors in human colon circular muscle: alterations in diverticular disease. J Pharmacol Exp Ther. 2002;302:627–35.
34. Simpson J, Sundler F, Jenkins D et al. Increased expression of substance P, neuropeptide K and galanin in mucosal nerves in patients with painful diverticular disease. Gastroenterology. 2004;126:A218.
35. Marrero JA, Matkowskyj KA, Yung K et al. Dextran sulfate sodium-induced murine colitis activates NF-kappaB and increases galanin-1 receptor expression. Am J Physiol Gastrointest Liver Physiol. 2000;278:G797–804.
36. Laird JM, Olivar T, Lopez-Garcia JA et al. Responses of rat spinal neurons to distension of inflamed colon: role of tachykinin NK2 receptors. Neuropharmacology. 2001;40:696–701.
37. Toulouse M, Coelho AM, Fioramonti J et al. Role of tachykinin NK2 receptors in normal and altered rectal sensitivity in rats. Br J Pharmacol. 2000;129:193–9.
38. Brandimarte G, Tursi A. Rifaximin plus mesalazine followed by mesalazine alone is highly effective in obtaining remission of symptomatic uncomplicated diverticular disease. Med Sci Monit. 2004;10:I70–3.

15
Determinants of treatment: extraintestinal comorbidity

B. LEMBCKE

INTRODUCTION

The scope of extraintestinal comorbidity in diverticular disease as a determinant of treatment may comprise genetic associations, unfavourable courses of diverticular disease as a sequel of lifestyle, of preexisting comorbidity or of environmental conditions, of therapy, and extraintestinal complications of diverticular disease.

Diverticular disease of the colon refers to three different conditions: (1) preferrably right-sided true diverticula, responsible for 70–75% of diverticulitis cases in Japan and Singapore; (2) weakness of connective tissue associated with pancolic diverticulosis and a tendency to bleed (e.g. in Marfan's syndrome); and (3) muscular hypertrophy of the left lower colon leading to diverticular disease with bleeding, diverticulitis and perforation as the typical complications.

According to the frame of this overview, the Asian variant of diverticulosis is not discussed further.

GENETIC ASSOCIATIONS

Epidemiology, time-course, and migration studies indicate that both the incidence and prevalence of diverticular disease are largely governed by environmental factors, e.g. nutrition (intake of dietary fibre), and physical activity. Subsequently, information about genetic associations of diverticular disease is sparse, especially with respect to treatment. While the Ehlers–Danlos syndrome may be associated with small bowel diverticula, no such association is reported for sigmoid diverticulosis. In Marfan's syndrome, however, both small and large bowel diverticula may complicate the clinical pattern[1,2].

Concerning the 'Western-type' of diverticular disease, a genetic linkage to (autosomal dominant) polycystic kidney disease (ADPKD) has been hypothesized from early clinical observations[3]. However, neither genetic chromosomal screening nor further clinical studies fostered a genetic linkage irrespective of an important clinical association of ADPKD and diverticular disease (see below).

POLYCYSTIC KIDNEY DISEASE

Scheff et al.[3] reported four patients with gross perforations due to diverticulitis among 12 of 151 haemodialysis patients (8%) having ADPKD, 10 of these 12 (83%) with colonic diverticulosis. Among 31 patients with chronic renal failure unrelated to ADPKD, n =10 (32%) had diverticulosis, none diverticulitis. Similarly, in a group of 120 age-matched non-renal failure control patients diverticulosis was diagnosed in 45 (38%) subjects, none of them had diverticulitis.

This report was corroborated by others. Lederman et al.[4] studied 184 patients with renal failure, 59 of them with polycystic kidney disease (group I). One hundred and twenty-five patients of this cohort had other causes of endstage renal disease (group II). Diverticulitis was observed in 12 (20%) of group I and four (3%) of group II ($p<0.003$). Moreover, six of the 12 patients with ADPKD and diverticulitis (50%) required surgical intervention. From the same institution it was shown that ADPKD accounted for 9% of the renal transplantation population but for 46% of the cases of diverticulitis ($p<0.001$) in this cohort[5].

Among 874 first renal transplant patients in Göteborg, 114 (13%) were transplanted for ADPKD. Studying these in more detail, and compared to 114 matched renal transplant control patients, a small but significant number of diverticulitis cases (4/114 vs 0/114; p = 0.03) was observed, two of them with perforation[6].

Other studies do not support a major role of diverticular disease in patients with polycystic kidney disease. Sharp et al.[7] identified 55 patients with ADPKD not receiving renal replacement therapy, and compared their barium enema results with two different controls, i.e. 12 unaffected family members and 59 random patients undergoing barium enemas (Table 1). Although absolute numbers are small, data do not support the view of a striking overexpression of diverticular disease in ADPKD which – *cum grano salis* – was present in approximately 50–60% of all study subjects at a mean age of 50 years. Similarly, Eigler's group from Essen[8] described a single (non-fatal) case of perforating sigmoid diverticulitis requiring surgery after renal transplantation for ADPKD among 46 patients (accounting for 4% of the total group of 1128 renal transplant patients) while 15 of 28 (54%) patients with polycystic kidney disease awaiting transplantation had colonic diverticulosis, one of them (without perforation) requiring surgery. These reports, although smaller in number, indicate that perforating diverticulitis might have been overemphasized earlier.

Today, the potentially dangerous course of diverticulitis in endstage renal disease (and transplantation as another immunocompromising condition) is well recognized[9] and, although not governed by evidence-based studies but guided by experience-based caution, sigmoid resection in patients with a history of true diverticulitis appears advisable if transplantation is planned. However, colonic screening prior to renal transplantation has only little impact on the post-transplantational course. The paper by McCune et al.[10] shows that the presence of diverticular disease in patients >50 years of age did not correspond to an increased incidence of diverticular complications after

Table 1 Differences in the prevalence and distribution of colonic diverticulosis cannot be responsible for a more aggressive course of diverticulitis complications in polycystic kidney disease (for explanations see text) (from ref. 7)

	Group I	*Group II*	*Group III*
Men	42%	42%	37%
Age (years)	49 ± 0.7	51 ± 2.1	49 ± 1
Diverticula	47%	58%	59%
Right colon	5%	17%	5%
Number	13.8	7.9	9.9

transplantation while perforating diverticulitis, if occurring, has an unfavourable course with a 40% mortality rate, irrespective of surgical therapy. On the basis of this experience from the Vanderbilt university (n = 1186 renal transplants) it no longer seemed warranted to screen asymptomatic patients >50 years of age for colonic diverticula. It is recommended, however, to screen those transplant candidates who had documented diverticulitis, who have ADPKD, or who report symptoms of diverticular disease.

Apparently, among endstage renal disease patients (ESRD), ADPKD patients do not die from associated diverticular disease but from cardiovascular or cerebrovascular disease. Overall mortality rate in ADPKD was lower than in the control group of non-diabetic ESRD[11].

ADPKD is the most common inherited kidney disease. It is genetically heterogeneous with mutations in two distinct genes leading to renal and liver cysts (AD-PKD1 corresponding to polycystin-1, an integral membrane protein that may serve as an extracellular receptor, and AD-PKD2 corresponding to polycystin-2, an integral membrane protein with characteristics of a calcium-permeant cation channel). A third gene (PKD3) is hypothesized but has not yet been identified. The genes responsible for *isolated* polycystic liver disease are different (PRKCSH; genetically linked to protein kinase C substrate 80K-H, encoding for hepatocystin, a protein that moderates glycosylation and fibroblast growth factor receptor signalling, and SEC63)[12–14].

Among the further conditions associated with the outcome of diverticular disease, the intake of non-steroidal anti-inflammatory drugs (NSAID) and obesity should be studied in more detail.

IMPACT OF NSAID

The wall of colonic diverticula consists predominantly of mucosa. Accordingly mechanisms impairing the mucosal barrier might be determinants or confounding factors of microperforation, which is the key process initiating diverticulitis and diverticular abscess formation.

NSAID may affect the mucosal barrier by altering microbial colonization, by altering mucin secretion, and by damage to epithelial cells[15–19].

Four case–control studies and a cohort study show an increased relative risk for complicated diverticular disease in diverticular disease patients taking

NSAIDS. Langman et al.[20], retrospectively reviewing 740 case records, described an association of perforation (large and small bowel) with NSAID use. Among the patients with perforation 22% took NSAID while this was the case in 10% only ($p<0.01$) of the control group with uncomplicated bowel disease.

The study by Corder[21] has more specifically addressed medication and diverticular perforation. Among 115 diverticular disease patients presenting with fistula, abscess and peritonitis NSAID use and corticosteroid use was more prevalent than in the 77 patients with diverticulitis and peridiverticulitis (i.e. without extracolonic sepsis). In this study NSAID use increased the relative risk for perforation by 4.9.

Wilson et al.[22] reported that bleeding and perforation, i.e. the major complications of diverticular disease was more likely to occur with NSAID if compared to an age- and sex-matched community-based control group (34% vs 4%, $p<0.001$) or to a group of colon cancer patients (34% vs 7%, $p<0.001$). Similar results were reported by Campbell et al.[23], who studied NSAID-associated morbidity in diverticular disease patients presenting with perforation and bleeding (n = 50) vs patients with emergency hospital admissions for other causes (n = 50), and patients with uncomplicated diverticular disease (n = 50). While in the first group 48% were taking NSAID, this was the case in 18% and 20%, respectively, of the control groups only.

A large cohort study in male health professionals by Aldoori et al.[24] suggests that regular and consistent use of NSAID in general, and acetaminophen, is associated with (self-reported) symptoms of diverticular disease, especially bleeding. While this is a large study and the design as a cohort study suggests more validity than case–control studies do, a critical editorial comment points out that criteria for diverticular symptoms in this study are weak and any event increasing the probability for a lower gastrointestinal diagnostic procedure will automatically increase the detection of diverticular disease, also if no causal relationship between diverticular disease and symptoms exist[25].

Reviewing the current understanding of the epidemiology of perforated colonic diverticular disease, however, Morris et al.[26] come to the conclusion that NSAID are identified as a consistent risk factor for complicating diverticular disease.

OBESITY

Obesity (frequent) is often associated with diverticular disease (also frequent), and obesity is generally accepted as a cause of diverticular disease, although this is not proven. However, obesity is an independent prognostic factor in perforated diverticular disease, and obesity has a measurable influence on the performance of elective laparoscopic colectomy in sigmoid diverticulitis.

Concerning the scenario of emergency operation for diverticulitis, Hansen and coworkers demonstrated by a multiple logistic regression model that preoperative sepsis syndrome (leucopenia and disturbed liver function), cardiac risk factors, and obesity are unfavourable prognostic factors in perforating diverticulitis. In different stages of diverticulitis (Hinchey I, 8.6%;

II, 14.3%; III, 57.1%; IV, 20%) mortality was 12.4%. With immunosuppression mortality rose to 33.3%. Using multivariate analysis, obesity significantly affected both mortality and local complications, while the increased mortality (21.4%) in obese patients did not gain statistical significance if tested along with univariate analysis ($p = 0.1$)[27].

Regarding mortality and morbidity after elective sigmoid resections for diverticulitis a recently published French multicenter trial with 582 elective sigmoid resections for diverticulitis[28] showed an operative mortality of 1.2% and an overall morbity of 24.9% (6.2% abdominal morbidity and 18.4% extraintestinal morbidity). Multivariate analysis revealed two significant independent risk factors (of 46 factors tested) for mortality, i.e. age >75 years (OR 7.9 (CI 1.7–36.6), $p = 0.01$), and obesity (BMI >30; OR 5.2 (CI 1.1–27.9), $p = 0.04$). Main risk factors for extra-abdominal morbidity were pulmonary disease (Pao_2 <65 mmHg) with an OR 2.9 (CI 1.4–6), $p = 0.008$, and liver cirrhosis (OR 1.2 (CI 1.2–120), $p = 0.02$),[28].

Another French study compared the results of laparoscopic sigmoid resection in 77 patients with normal weight (BMI 18–24.9; group I), overweight (BMI 25–29.9; group II), and obesity (BMI 30–39.9; group III). There were no differences concerning age, sex, ASA classification, or postoperative hospital stay. Mortality was nil in all groups, and morbidity was 15%, 14%, and 17%, respectively (n.s.). Similarly, conversion rates were not different. However, there was a significantly longer duration of operation (247 min vs 187 min) and a longer need for parenteral analgetics (8.5 days vs 5.7 days) in group III vs group I[29].

Data from the Cleveland Clinic, Florida, strongly foster the view that obese patients undergoing laparoscopic colorectal surgery have higher conversion rates and a significantly higher risk concerning postoperative complications, ileus, wound infections, and hospital stay (Table 2)[30].

Obesity is further corroborated as an independent risk factor for wound infections in another study on complications of elective colorectal surgery[31]. As in the study by Wexner's group[30] these data were obtained in patients with different aetiologies of colorectal disease. Along with severe adhesions and colonic inflammation, obesity is reported as a major cause for conversion in another multicentre study in 179 patients undergoing elective laparoscopic colonic resection for diverticular disease[32].

Table 2 Obesity as a complicating factor for elective laparoscopic segmental colonic resections (various indications for surgery) (from ref. 30)

	Obese (BMI >30) n = 31 (19.1%)	*Non-obese n = 131*	*p-Value*
Conversion rate	39%	13.5%	0.01
Postoperative complications	78%	24%	0.01
Ileus	32.3%	7.6%	0.01
Wound infection	12.9%	3.1%	0.03
Hospital stay (days)	9.5	6.9	0.02

EXTRAINTESTINAL COMPLICATIONS

Another aspect of extraintestinal comorbidity with therapeutic implications are pyogenic complications which originate from (micro)perforation. Fistulas or local abscesses of the sigmoid colon may drain towards the urinary bladder (most often in men) or towards the vagina, thus leading to pneumaturia or genitourinary infections (Figure 1). Diverticular disease is the predominant aetiology of colovesical fistulas (> Crohn's disease > carcinoma) with faecaluria, abdominal pain, and pneumaturia as the commonest presenting symptoms[33,34]. Again, in the immunocompromised patient, colovesical fistula and recurrent (graft) pyelonephritis may occur with silent diverticulitis[35]. While cystoscopy is of major value for the diagnosis of a colovesical fistula, sigmoidoscopy is less accurate than barium enema or computed tomography (CT) and ultrasonography. The latter are also guiding examinations in patients with chronic recurrent sigmoid inflammation leading to a conglomerate tumour as a cause of ureter stenosis with subsequent left-sided hydronephrosis. In both these situations elective surgery is the therapy of choice[33–35].

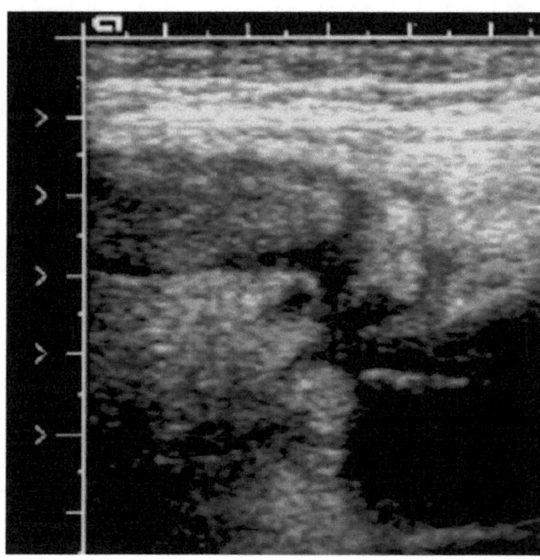

Figure 1 Colovesical fistula at ultrasonography (Accuson 128)

Ascending infection via the mesenteric veins may give rise to pyephlebitis of the portal vein and, finally, pyogenic hepatic abscess (Figure 2). While antibiotic therapy of diverticulitis concurrently implies the rational antibiotic treatment for pyephlebitis, thrombotic obliteration with portal hypertension may ensue during healing. Whether or not a therapeutically prolonged partial prothrombin time (PTT) really prevents portal vein thrombosis or reduces the

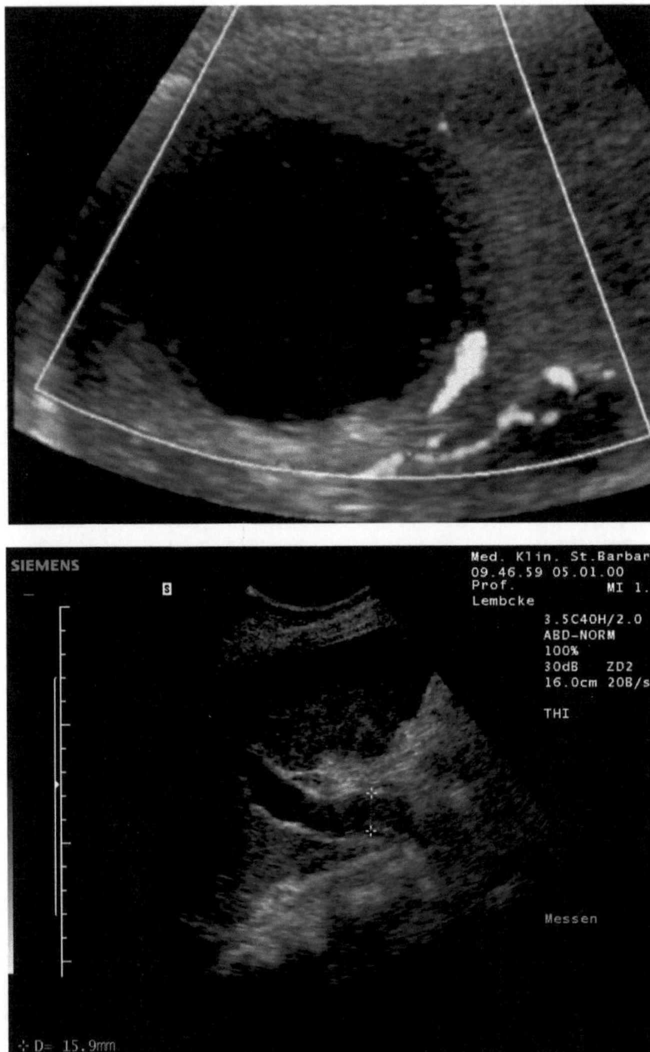

A

B

Figure 2 Pyogenic hepatic abscess (**A**) and underlying pyephlebitis of the portal vein (**B**) as extraintestinal septic complications of diverticulitis at ultrasonography (Siemens Elegra)

rate of remaining obliteration in this scenario, is not clear, but full heparinization is routinely performed.

In the case of pyogenic liver abscess, however, additional percutaneous ultrasound-guided (or CT-guided) drainage is sometimes mandatory (larger pyogenic mass, rapid enlargement, risk of rupture). Interventional drainage of hepatic abscess is performed either by direct puncture with an 8–10F catheter or by a Seldinger technique followed by step-by-step dilation of the canal and stable insertion of a 12–14F drainage catheter. The same procedure may be used (a) as a definitive therapy for the drainage of localized, single, easily accessible paracolic abscesses (Hinchey I, II) along with a conservative regimen; and (b) as a bridging, stabilizing intervention in the context of a local accessible large abscess in a difficult situation (e.g. sepsis, comorbidity). Phlegmoneous inflammation is no indication for interventional drainage, and the aspiration of faeculent material will certainly prevent success of percutaneous drainage.

As in other situations with a protracted and severe course of gastrointestinal infection and/or an intensive care approach, endogenous *Candida* endophthalmitis has been described as a rare but devastating complication, usually requiring intensive and early antimycotic therapy as well as early vitrectomy. Prognosis, however, is usually poor[36].

Anecdotally, arthritis is reported as an extra-intestinal manifestation of diverticulitis[37]. Current understanding is that this is related to autoimmunity (enteric arthritis) rather than to a septic bacterial spread. In a well-documented case arthritis did not respond to medical therapy (while diverticulitis did), but it improved after resection of the sigmoid colon[37].

TRANSPLANTATION

Transplant immunosuppression gives rise to a number of gastrointestinal complications (e.g. cytomegalovirus (CMV) infections, bacterial complications, e.g. pseudomembranous colitis; perforations; ischaemia and malignancy) and, among these, diverticulitis plays a significant role, irrespective of the organ transplanted[38–41].

Renal transplantation

Not unexpectedly most experience with diverticulitis exists in renal transplant patients. The rate of colonic perforations due to diverticulitis in major retrospective studies accounts for approximately 0.6–0.9% (Table 3)[5,8,42–45]. Complicated diverticulitis in the transplant patient may occur both early after transplantation (75% in the first 3 months), and years thereafter. The incidence and outcome of post-transplant perforation are associated with the intensity of immunosuppression, the mean daily corticosteroid dose being three times higher in those patients who died than in the survivors, while neither cyclosporin nor donor source seem to play a major role for perforating diverticulitis occurrence[5,43]. Furthermore, poor nutritional status, as indicated by low albumin levels, is a risk factor for not surviving in this situation[43]. Early

Table 3 Severe colonic (diverticulitis) complications after renal transplantation

Reference	*Transplant patients*	*Colonic perforations*	*Origin*
Soravia et al.[42]	2091	12 (9) (0.5%)	Belgium
Stelzner et al.[43]	1401	30 (2.1%)	Boston
Pirenne et al.[44]	1530	8 (0.5%)	Minnesota
Dominguez et al.[8]	1128	1 (0.1%)	Essen
Lederman et al.[5]	1137	13 (1.1%)	New York

Table 4 Severe diverticulitis after heart and lung transplantation

Type of transplant and reference	*Transplant patients*	*Colonic perforations*	*Origin*
Lung[48]	66	4 (6.6%)	Denver
Lung[49]	35	3 (8.6%)	Gainesville
Heart[50]	143	6 (4%)	Liege (B)
Heart and lung[51]	268	2 (0.7%)	Detroit
Heart, lung, heart/lung[52]	953	9 (1%)	Sydney

colonic perforations are mainly attributed to heavy immunosuppression and ongoing dialysis, leading to diverticulitis and CMV colitis-induced perforations, whereas late perforations are mainly attributed to diverticulosis and malignancy (e.g. lymphoma)[40]. Late intra-abdominal abscess formation due to unexpected diverticulitis has also been reported in rather young patients with renal transplantation (one teenager and one in the mid-20s)[46].

Colonic ulcerations have been described as an occasional side-effect of mycophenolate mofetil[47].

Heart and lung transplantation

Following heart or lung or combined heart–lung transplantations the incidence of colonic perforations appears to be significantly higher than reported in renal transplants (Table 4)[48–52]. While data from Detroit and Sydney in rather larger series indicate complicated diverticulitis in 0.7% and 1.0%[51,52], respectively, reports from smaller series of thoracic transplant recipients emphasize substantially higher rates of perforations[48–50]. There is no evident reason for this discrepancy; however, two impressions might be noteworthy. First, the series with lower diverticulitis perforations have been reported 4-8 years later. Secondly, these reports[51,52] reflect the situation from experienced institutions of colorectal surgery while the other reports originate from cardiovascular surgery or medical institutions[48–50] with potentially different, more corticosteroid-based immunosuppressive regimens in the postoperative phase. Overall, the incidence of acute diverticulitis-related colonic perforations with

1.6% in the thoracic transplant recipients is twice as high as in the renal transplant recipients. Concerning the risk of perforating diverticulitis in thoracic transplant recipients versus the non-transplanted population, the data of Qasabian et al.[52] demonstrate a 22.2-fold increase (CI 9.9–50.0; $p < 0.001$) after heart transplant/liver transplant.

The supposedly higher cardiopulmonary stress due to haemodynamis changes in accompanying pneumoperitoneum has not raised complications in two heart transplant patients with acute diverticulitis without perforation or peritonitis, who underwent laparoscopic-assisted colectomy[53].

WHAT MATTERS ?

Age, obesity, sepsis, severe immunosuppression, reduced nutritional status and NSAID medication play a considerable role for diverticulitis complications and outcome. Local and septic complications, e.g. left-sided hydronephosis, genito-urinary fistulas or pyogenic pyephlebitis and liver abscess, deserve diagnostic attention. Enterogenic arthritis or metastatic fungal infections are rare. Patients with polycystic kidney disease, and transplanted patients, deserve special considerations. In diverticulitis patients, extraintestinal comorbidity requires extraordinary cooperation between gastroenterologists and surgeons. Especially in the situation of the transplanted patient their expertise is reflected by a high index of suspicion and a low threshold for operation.

References

1. Clunie GJA, Mason JM. Visceral diverticula and the Marfan syndrome. Br J Surg. 1962;50:51–2.
2. Harendra de Silva DG, Gunawardena TPJ, Law FMK. Unusual complications in siblings with marfanoid phenotype. Arch Dis Child. 1996;75:247–8.
3. Scheff RT, Zuckerman G, Harter H, Delmez J, Koehler R. Diverticular disease in patients with chronic renal failure due to polycystic kidney disease. Ann Intern Med. 1980;92:202–4.
4. Lederman ED, McCoy G, Conti DJ, Lee EC. Diverticulitis and polycystic kidney disease. Am Surg. 2000;66:200–3.
5. Lederman ED, Conti DJ, Lempert N, Sigh TP, Lee EC. Complicated diverticulitis following renal transplantation. Dis Colon Rectum. 1998;41:613–18.
6. Hadimeri H, Nordén G, Friman S, Nyberg G. Autosomal dominant polycystic kidney disease in a kidney transplant population. Nephrol Dial Transplant. 1997;12:1431–6.
7. Sharp CK, Zeligman BE, Johnson AM, Duley I, Gabow PA. Evaluation of colonic diverticular disease in autosomal dominant polycystic kidney disease without end-stage renal disease. Am J Kidney Dis. 1999;34:863–8.
8. Dominguez Fernandez E, Albrecht KH, Heemann U et al. Prevalence of diverticulosis and incidence of bowel perforation after kidney transplantation in patients with polycystic kidney disease. Transplant Int. 1998;11:28–31.
9. Starnes HF Jr, Lazarus JM, Vineyard G. Surgery for diverticulitis in renal failure. Dis Colon Rectum. 1985;28:827–31.
10. McCune TR, Nylander WA, Van Buren DH et al. Colonic screening prior to renal transplantation and its impact on post-transplant colonic complications. Clin Transplant. 1992;6:91–6.
11. Perrone RD, Ruthazer R, Terrin NC. Survival after end-stage renal disease in autosomal dominant polycystic kidney disease: contribution of extrarenal complications to mortality. Am J Kidney Dis. 2001;38:777–84.

12. Wilson PD. Polycystic kidney disease. N Engl J Med. 2004;350:151–64.
13. Everson GT, Taylor MR, Doctor RB. Polycystic disease of the liver. Hepatology. 2004;40:774–82.
14. Everson GT, Taylor MR. Management of polycystic liver disease. Curr Gastroenterol Rep. 2005;7:19–25.
15. Levi S, Shaw-Smith C. Non-steroidal anti-inflammatory drugs: how do they damage the gut ? Br J Rheumatol. 1994;33:605–12.
16. Davies NM, Wallace JL. Nonsteroidal anti-inflammatory drug-induced gastrointestinal toxicity: new insights into an old problem. J Gastroenterol. 1997;32:127–33.
17. Cryer B. NSAID gastrointestinal toxicity. Curr Opin Gastroenterol. 2000;16:495–502.
18. Davies NM. Toxicity of nonsteroidal anti-inflammatory drugs in the large intestine. Dis Colon Rectum. 1995;38:1311–21.
19. Davies NM. Review article: Non-steroidal anti-inflammatory drug-induced gastrointestinal permeability. Aliment Pharmacol Ther. 1998;12:303–20.
20. Langman MJ, Morgan L, Worrall A. Use of anti-inflammatory drugs by patients admitted with small and large bowel perforations and haemorrhage. Br Med J. 1985;290:347–9.
21. Corder A. Steroids, non-steroidal anti-inflammatory drugs, and serious septic complications of diverticular disease. Br Med J. 1987;295:1238.
22. Wilson RG, Smith AN, MacIntyre IM. Complications of diverticular disease and non-steroidal anti-inflammatory drugs: a prospective study. Br J Surg. 1990;77:1103–4.
23. Campbell K, Steele RJ. Non-steroidal anti-inflammatory drugs and complicated diverticular disease: a case–control study. Br J Surg. 1991;78:190–1.
24. Aldoori WH, Giovannucci EL, Rimm EB, Wing AL, Willett WC. Use of acetaminophen and nonsteroidal anti-inflammatory drugs. A prospective study and the risk of symptomatic diverticular disease in men. Arch Fam Med. 1998;7:255–60.
25. Mold JW (editorial). Analgesics and symptomatic diverticular disease. Arch Fam Med. 1998;7:262–3.
26. Morris CR, Harvey IM, Stebbings WSL, Speakman CTM, Kennedy HJ, Hart AR. Epidemiology of perforated colonic diverticular disease. Postgrad Med J. 2002;78:654–9.
27. Hansen O, Graupe F, Stock W. Prognosefaktoren der perforierteen dickdarmdiverticulitis. Chirurg 1998;69:443–9.
28. Pessaux P, Muscari F, Ouellet JF et al., French Association for Surgical Research. Risk factors for mortality and morbidity after elective sigmoid resection for diverticulitis: prospective multicenter multivariate analysis of 582 patients. World J Surg. 2004;28:92–6.
29. Tuech JJ, Regenet N, Hennekinne S. Pessaux P, Berggamschi R, Arnaud JP. Laparoscopic colectomy for sigmoid diverticulitis in obese and nonobese patients: a prospective comparative study. Surg Endosc. 2001;15:1427–30.
(idem: Tuech JJ, Regenet N, Hennekinne S. Pessaux P, Duplessis R, Arnaud JP. Impact of obesity on postoperative results of elective laparoscopic colectomy in sigmoid diverticulitis: a prospective study [in French]. Ann Chir. 2001;126:996–1000)
30. Pikarsky AJ, Saida Y, Yamaguchi T et al. Is obesity a high-risk factor for laparoscopic colorectal surgery? Surg Endosc. 2002;16:855–8.
31. Smith RL, Bohl JK, McElearney ST et al. Wound infection after elective colorectal resection. Ann Surg. 2004;239:599–607.
32. Bouillot JL, Berthou JC, Champault G et al. Elective laparoscopic colonic resection for diverticular disease: results of a multicenter study in 179 patients. Surg Endosc. 2002;16:1320–3.
33. Hafner CD, Ponka JL, Brush BE. Genitourinary manifestations of diverticulitis of the colon: a study of 5000 cases. J Am Med Assoc. 1962;179:174–6.
34. Kirsh GM, Hampel N, Shuck JM, Resnick MI. Diagnosis and management of vesicoenteric fistulas. Surg Gynecol Obstet. 1991;173;91–7.
35. Rodrigo E, Ruiz JC, L^{4}pez-Rasines G et al. Recurrent graft pyelonephritis and pneumaturia resulting from a colovesical fistula secondary to silent diverticulitis. Nephrol Dial Transplant 1998;13:1001–3.
36. Stoffelns BM. Endogenous *Candida* endophthalmitis combined with severe deneral disease (German). Klin Monatsbl Augenheilkd. 2005;222:214–17.
37. Alba S, Nascimbeni R, DiBetta E, Villanacci V, Salerni B. Arthritis as a rare extra-intestinal manifestation of acute sigmoid diverticulitis. Dig Surg. 2001;18:233–4.

38. Mona D, Largiader F, Binswanger U, Sulser H. Colonic complications after renal transplantation [German]. Langenbecks Arch Chir. 1982;357:141–50.
39. Lao A, Bach D. Colonic complications in renal transplant patients. Dis Colon Rectum. 1988;31:130–3.
40. Helderman JH, Goral S. Gastrointestinal complications of transplant immunosuppression. J Am Soc Nephrol. 2002;13:277–87.
41. Maurer JR. The spectrum of colonic complications in a lung transplant population. Ann Transplant 2000;5:54–7.
42. Soravia C, Baldi A, Kartheuser A et al. Acute colonic complications after kidney transplantation. Acta Chir Belg. 1995;95:157–61.
43. Stelzner M, Vlahakos DV, Milford EL, Tilney NL. Colonic perforations after renal transplantation. J Am Coll Surg. 1997;184:63–9.
44. Pirenne J, Lledo-Garcia E, Benedetti E et al. Colonic perforation after renal transplantation: a single-institution review. Clin Transplant. 1997;11:88–93.
45. Flanigan RC, Reckard CR, Lucas BA. Colonic complications of renal transplantation. J Urol. 1988;139;503–6.
46. Abramson SJ, Berdon WE, Laffey K, Ruzal-Shapiro C, Nash M, Baer J. Colonic diverticulitis in young patients with chronic renal failure and transplantation. Pediatr Radiol. 1991;21:352–4.
47. Galconda M, Valente J, Bejarano P, Gilinsky N, First MR. Colonic ulceration. A previously unreported adverse effect of mycophenolate mofetil. Transplantation. 1998;65(Suppl.):224 (Abstract).
48. Beaver TM, Fullerton DA, Zamora MR et al. Colon perforation after lung transplantation. Ann Thorac Surg. 1996;62:839–43.
49. Fenton JJ, Cicale MJ. Sigmoid diverticular perforation complicating lung transplantation. J Heart Lung Transplant. 1997;16:681–5.
50. Detry O, Defraigne JO, Meurisse M et al. Acute diverticulitis in heart transplant recipients. Transplant Int. 1996;9:376–9.
51. Khan S, Eppstein AC, Anderson GK et al. Acute diverticulitis in heart- and lung-transplant patients. Transplant Int. 2001;14:12–15.
52. Qasabian RA, Meagher AP, Lee R, Dore GJ, Keogh A. Severe diverticulitis after heart, lung, and heart–lung transplantation. J Heart Lung Transplant. 2004;23:845–9.
53. Detry O, Defraigne JO, Chiche JD et al. Laparoscopic-assisted colectomy in heart transplant recipients. Clin Transplant. 1996;10:191–4.

16
Determinants of treatment: outcome measures, or how to read studies on diverticulitis

J. C. HOFFMANN and M. ZEITZ

INTRODUCTION

As in other diseases, doctors try to treat diverticular disease patients with the most effective and least harmful treatment at the lowest cost. Consequently, prevention would be the preferred management followed by effective conservative treatment. In contrast, invasive treatment, e.g. drainage and/or surgery, has the least favourable profile and needs to be avoided unless good evidence exists that shows a better outcome than conservative treatment. Once diverticulitis has occurred, only medical or interventional treatment modalities remain. In order to develop treatment recommendations for the individual patient the existing studies need to be carefully analysed, aiming at the development of evidence-based guidelines if at all possible. Prior to that, however, one has to consider whether published studies are comparable with each other and whether they have used similar or even identical diagnostic criteria as well as classification systems. In addition, already-published guidelines by the American Society of Colorectal Surgeons (ASCRS), the practice guidelines by the American College of Gastroenterology (ACG), and the European Consensus Report on diagnosis and treatment of diverticular disease (European Association for Endoscopic Surgery, EAES) should be looked at with regard to the validity of their recommendations[1–4]. Finally, one should keep in mind that the measurement of diverticulitis outcome has limitations that cannot be overcome. For instance, it is sometimes difficult to distinguish whether a complication postoperatively is surgery- or disease-related, e.g. a fistula. Persistence of symptoms, e.g. abdominal pain, can also be multifactorial.

Diverticular disease can be divided into three entities: diverticulitis, diverticular bleeding, and symptomatic diverticulosis. This chapter will focus on diverticulitis since diverticulitis is the subgroup of diverticular disease that represents the most important inpatient subgroup combined with the largest number of available studies.

DEFINITIONS, DIAGNOSTIC CRITERIA, CLASSIFICATION SYSTEMS

Diverticulitis is defined as inflammation of diverticula. While typical symptoms such as left-sided lower abdominal pain, fever, and a mass on physical examination are well-known findings in diverticulitis, no international definition exists as to what is required for a clear diagnosis of diverticulitis. In general, diagnostic criteria are not needed for daily practice, but would be extremely helpful when one wants to compare results from different studies. So far published studies have used different criteria for defining diverticulitis and its recurrence; some examples are shown in Table 1. These demonstrate that

Table 1 Study definition on diverticulitis

Author (year)	*Definition*
Horner (1952)[16]	Required symptoms: constipation/diarrhoea, cramping, tenderness, fever, leucocytosis
Zollinger (1968)[7]	'Adequate past history tabulated in the hospital records'
Parks (1969)[5]	Clinical features, together with (a) radiological or (b) pathological evidence
Tudor et al. (1994)[8]	'Considered on clinical grounds to have complicated diverticulitis'
Elliot et al. (1997)[9]	ICD 9 diagnosis

even recent studies have used very soft inclusion criteria, e.g. by stating that patients with the ICD9 discharge diagnosis of diverticulitis were included. Studies on subgroups or studies on different treatement modalities have the drawback that other illnesses can mimic diverticulitis or its recurrence, e.g. irritable bowel syndrome. For instance, the excellent study by Parks from 1969 used persistent or recurrent abdominal pain as sufficient evidence for the definition of persistent or recurrent diverticulitis[5]. Therefore, we need diagnostic criteria that use non-invasive methods in order to objectively diagnose diverticulitis without requiring a surgical specimen. While ultrasound has a sensitivity and specificity similar to computed tomography (CT) scanning it is more difficult to verify the presence of diverticulitis on videos or pictures. Therefore, diagnostic criteria for future studies on diverticulitis are urgently needed and, most probably, will require a CT scan. In spite of its radiation a CT scan is also required for patients with recurrence unless severe complications have occurred that require immediate surgery.

Looking at the pathological spectrum of diverticulitis it is evident that some patients are less, and others are more, severly affected. These differences are reflected when we talk about complicated and non-complicated diverticulitis. Unfortunately, much controversy exists regarding the definition of complicated diverticulitis. Clearly, faecal peritonitis because of perforation is complicated, but it is less clear whether peridiverticulitis is complicated or non-complicated. Classification systems shown in Table 2 are of help[10–15]. All these classification systems have advantages and disadvantages; however, it is of the utmost importance to look carefully at the definition of 'complicated diverticulitis' when one wants to compare different studies which deal with 'complicated diverticulitis'. For instance Hansen[10] defines peridiverticulitis as complicated while many others do not.

Table 2 Classification system

Findings	*Hansen*	*Siewert*	*Hinchey*	*Hughes*	*Sher*	*Ambrosetti*
Diverticulosis	0					
Acute uncomplicated diverticulitis	I					Mild
Peridiverticulitis, phlegmon	IIa	I		I		Moderate
Abscess (pericolic, mesocolic)	IIa	I	I	II	I	Severe
Pelvic abscess	IIb	II	II	II	IIa	Severe
Free perforation, purulent peritonitis	IIc	III	III	III	III	Severe
Free perforation, faecal peritonitis	IIc	III	IV	IV	IV	Severe
Recurrent diverticulitis, fistula	III				IIb	

DRAWBACKS OF PUBLISHED GUIDELINES

Overall, four clinical guidelines have been published: one practice guideline by the American College of Gastroenterology (ACG), one guideline by the American Society of Colon and Rectal Surgeons (ASCRS) orginally published in 1995 and in revised form in 2000, one therapeutic guideline on acute right colonic diverticulitis from Japan, and one consensus statement of a Scientific Committee of the European Association of Endoscopic Surgery (EAES) on the diagnosis and treatment of diverticular disease[1–4,16]. Only the EAES guideline was developed in a formal consensus process, although with some limitations; for instance, the published evidence was reported only for certain aspects of the topic. The Japanese guideline is in fact a report on right-sided diverticulitis rather than a clinical guideline. As mentioned above, there is no general agreement concerning the definition of complicated diverticulitis. While the ACG guideline does not even define complicated diverticulitis, the ASCRS guideline excludes, and the EAES guideline includes, phlegmon as a complication. Since peridiverticulitis and phlegmon are probably the most common subtypes of diverticulitis that present to emergency departments this is an important difference; it illustrates that we need an internationally accepted definition of complicated diverticulitis or, even better, an internationally accepted classification system including diagnostic criteria.

Apart from this important difference concerning the definition of complicated diverticulitis the guidelines agree on two important aspects concerning the management of diverticulitis: the indication for elective surgery in young patients (after the first attack) and upon recurrence (after the second attack). These important recommendations have recently been questioned by two groups, one performing a model decision analysis (Markov model) based on a population-based database, and the other one reviewing the published evidence for these recommendations[17,18]. With regard to the recommendation concerning elective surgery for recurrent diverticulitis three studies are usually cited, one retrospective analysis by Parks from 1969[5], second a study by Farmakis et al. using a prospective cohort[19], and third the original ASCRS guideline[1]. All three studies state that the complications and the mortality rate are increased after the second attack of diverticulitis. If one looks in further detail into these studies major problems become evident:

1. The 1995 ASCRS guideline does not give data substantiating the recommendation of surgery after the second attack.

2. The study by Parks was not only retrospective but also included patients with abdominal pain and radiological evidence of diverticulosis rather than diverticulitis as defined by intraoperative, postmortem or CT scanning findings. Further, the reason for initial operation or against operation was not defined. Therefore, it is possible that patients with complicated diverticulitis were not intially operated upon because of comorbidity. Finally, recurrence and/or persistence of diverticulitis was defined by the presence of abdominal pain. Clearly, some patients with diverticulosis have irritable bowel syndrome rather than persistent or reccurrent diverticulitis.

3. The study by Farmakis and co-workers reporting on the natural history of complicated diverticular disease was based on a prospective cohort of patients as originally published by Tudor et al.[8]. The most important statement in this paper was that 'only two of 77 patients who had initially been managed by resection compared to 37 of 43 managed conservatively developed recurrent complications'. In this study nine patients after conservative treatment, and only one after resection, died because of diverticulitis. Although this study was prospective no criteria were given as to why patients were initially managed conservatively. This study included phlegmon as complicated diverticulitis. However, phlegmon was defined as 'left iliac fossa mass without fever'. It is well known that an abscess does not always lead to fever; therefore it is unclear how many patients with an abscess but without fever (here called phlegmon) should have had an operation in the first place. In addition, the data concerning the course after the initial episode of diverticulitis were based on a questionnaire dispatched to general practitoners (GP). One might ask how often the GP had good evidence for the assumption that his/her patient died because of complicated diverticular disease.

Taken together, the recommendation for elective surgery after the second attack is not based on solid ground. Recently, a population-based study showed that the adjusted hazard ratio for emergency colectomy/colostomy was increased after the second episode and also increased among patients younger than 50 years of age[20]. However, only 7.5% of young patients required emergency operation and a model decision analysis by the same group revealed that performing colectomy after the fourth rather than the second episode in patients older than 50 years resulted in 0.5% fewer deaths, 0.7% fewer colostomies, and saved $1035 while in younger patients the values were 0.1% fewer deaths, 2% fewer colostomies and $5429 saved per patient when comparing an operation after the fourth rather than the first episode[17]. Therefore, most recent evidence suggests that current guidelines are not evidence-based, and that the guidelines should be revised with regard to recommendations for the indications for elective surgery.

OUTCOME MEASURES: DISEASE-RELATED, TREATMENT-RELATED

Apart from the above-mentioned problems concerning the definition of complicated diverticulitis, and concerning important aspects of current guidelines, clinical studies on diverticulitis lack uniform measures of outcome such as an activity index. In general, outcome measures can be subdivided into morbidity-, mortality-, and cost-related. In addition, these measures can either be disease- or treatment-related. Treatment-related factors depend on the type of treatment, i.e. complications after conservative treatment, complications related to surgery, and complications related to anaesthesia. An example for such a classification is shown in Table 3.

ECONOMIC CONSIDERATIONS

Only a few reports have been published on costs for diverticular disease. Delvau calculated that, for the 'old' European countries with a population of 376 million people, 102 million people would have diverticulosis, giving about 60 000 perforations/year (estimated incidence 16/100 000), 786 000 hospital admissions (estimated incidence 209/100 000), and 23 000 deaths from diverticular disease (estimated mortality rate 3%)[21]. If one calculates further

Table 3 Classification of treatment-related morbitiy

Conservative treatment
Antibiotic-associated complications (e.g. pseudomembranous colitis)
General complications (e.g. deep venous thrombosis, pulmonary embolism)
Recurrence in high-risk groups (e.g. immunosuppression)
Sepsis
Operative treatment: anaesthesia-related
Respiratory failure, pneumonia
General complications (e.g. catheter sepsis, pneumonia, pneumothorax)
Operative treatment: surgery-related
Anastomotic leakage
Uncontrolled sepsis
Bleeding, wound infections, incisional hernia
Fistula
Abscess

that about 25% will be operated upon for 5000 Euros per patient, the annual total costs for surgery almost 1 billion Euros per year. Conservative treatment is less expensive, and can be estimated to cost about 2500 Euros per patient, making almost 1.5 billion Euros for conservative treatment per year. As mentioned above, a recent model decision analysis suggests that money could be saved, combined with reduced morbidity and mortality, if elective surgery for uncomplicated diverticulitis (including peridiverticulitis and phlegmon) were postponed[13].

CONCLUSIONS

Diverticular disease, particularly diverticulitis, is an economically important disease. So far agreement on the definition of complicated diverticulitis, as well as an internationally accepted classification system, are missing. These would be very important for the comparison of different clinical trials. With regard to current clinical guidelines, recommending elective colon resection after the second attack of uncomplicated diverticulitis (including peridiverticulitis and phlegmon), or even after the first attack if the patient is less than 50 years of age, is not evidence-based. Future revisions hopefully will change these recommendations. Finally, clinical studies would benefit from a diverticulitis disease activity index. Unfortunately, such an index is not available at present.

References

1. Roberts P, Abel M, Rosen L et al. Practice parameters for sigmoid diverticulitis. Standards Task Force American Society of Colon and Rectal Surgeons. Dis Colon Rectum. 1995;38: 125–32.
2. Stollman NH, Raskin JB. Diverticular disease of the colon. J Clin Gastroenterol. 1999;29: 241–52.
3. Kohler L, Sauerland S, Neugebauer E. Diagnosis and treatment of diverticular disease: results of a consensus development conference. Scientific Committee of the European Association for Endoscopic Surgery. Surg Endosc. 1999;13:430–6.
4. Wong WD, Wexner SD, Lowry A et al. Practice parameters for the treatment of sigmoid diverticulitis – supporting documentation. Standards Task Force. The American Society of Colon and Rectal Surgeons. Dis Colon Rectum. 2000;43:290–7.
5. Parks TG. Natural history of diverticular disease of the colon. A review of 521 cases. Br Med J. 1969;4:639–42.
6. Horner JL. A study of diverticulitis of the colon in office practice. Gastroenterology. 1952;21:223–9.
7. Zollinger RW. The prognosis in diverticulitis of the colon. Arch Surg. 1968;97:418–22.
8. Tudor RG, Farmakis N, Keighley MR. National audit of complicated diverticular disease: analysis of index cases. Br J Surg. 1994;81:730–2.
9. Elliott TB, Yego S, Irvin TT. Five-year audit of the acute complications of diverticular disease. Br J Surg. 1997;84:535–9.
10. Hansen OS. Prophylaktische Operation bei der Divertikelkrankheit des Kolon-stufenkonzeptes durch exakte Stadieneinteilung. Langenbecks Arch Surg. 1999;II:1257.
11. Siewert JR, Huber FT, Brune IB. Frühe elektive Chirurgie der akuten Divertikulitis des Colons. Chirurg. 1995;66:1182–9.
12. Hinchey EJ, Schaal PG, Richards GK. Treatment of perforated diverticular disease of the colon. Adv Surg. 1978;12:85–109.
13. Hughes ES, Cuthbertson AM, Carden AB. The surgical management of acute diverticulitis. Med J Austr. 1963;50:780–2.

14. Sher ME, Agachan F, Bortul M, Nogueras JJ, Weiss EG, Wexner SD. Laparoscopic surgery for diverticulitis. Surg Endosc. 1997;11:264–7.
15. Ambrosetti P, Becker C, Terrier F. Colonic diverticulitis: impact of imaging on surgical management – a prospective study of 542 patients. Eur Radiol. 2002;12:1145–9.
16. Komuta K, Yamanaka S, Okada K et al. Toward therapeutic guidelines for patients with acute right colonic diverticulitis. Am J Surg. 2004;187:233–7.
17. Salem L, Veenstra DL, Sullivan SD, Flum DR. The timing of elective colectomy in diverticulitis: a decision analysis. J Am Coll Surg. 2004;199:904–12.
18. Janes S, Meagher A, Frizelle FA. Elective surgery after acute diverticulitis. Br J Surg. 2005; 92:133–42.
19. Farmakis N, Tudor RG, Keighley MR. The 5-year natural history of complicated diverticular disease. Br J Surg. 1994;81:733–5.
20. Anaya DA, Flum DR. Assessing the risk of emergency colectomy and colostomy in patients with diverticular disease. Arch Surg. 2005;40:681–5.
21. Delvaux M. Diverticular disease of the colon in Europe: epidemiology, impact on citizen health and prevention. Aliment Pharmacol Ther. 2003;18(Suppl. 3):71–4.

Section VII
Surgery

Chair: W. FLEIG and S. WEXNER

17
Extent of sigmoid resection in diverticular disease of the colon

A. FINGERHUT and R. BERGAMASCHI

INTRODUCTION

The question of the length of the resected segment when performing colectomy for diverticular disease of the colon is certainly not new. However, interest in this topic has recently been renewed and reviewed. The site of anastomosis, the length of the specimen, as well as the extent of mesenteric resection, have all been thought to be important determinants of the recurrence rate, the safety of the anastomosis, and satisfactory patient comfort. While the level of evidence for most of the recommendations provided by the authors' research of the literature is not high, a great deal of information, based on time-proven experience, is available.

Although diverticula can exist in almost any portion of the digestive tract, most are found in the left colon, and in particular, in the sigmoid colon[1]. The indications for resection have been dealt with elsewhere in this volume and will not be discussed here. For the remainder of this chapter, we will deal with resection of the sigmoid colon unless specified otherwise.

Several studies[2–10] have looked at the appropriate length of resection and the site of anastomosis in the specific setting of elective resection.

In the elective setting, resection of the entire sigmoid colon has been the modern standard since Judd's publications from the Mayo Clinic[2,3] in 1955 and 1962, in which it was found that, even when diverticula were present in the transverse or right colons, the sigmoid colon was the site of the severe complications in over 98% of patients. While this theory is more or less the rule for most surgeons, there is still some ongoing debate as to the reasons for defining the upper (and lower) limits of colonic resection for diverticular disease. The extent of resection may also differ somewhat according to whether the operation is performed in the elective or emergency settings, and in the latter, in the case of haemorrhage, whether the diverticula responsible for bleeding have been located or not.

Bergamaschi and Arnaud[5], in their discussion, cited a paper from Munson et al.[6] for the recommendation of resecting all visibly involved colonic segments in order to achieve a safe anastomosis in a portion of the colon without diverticula or inflammation. The paper by Munson et al.[6], however, gave no details as to the histology of the resection margins. Other authors[4,7] have debated the oral limit of resection, without being able to come to any formal conclusions[1]. Bergamaschi and Arnaud[5] provide us, however, with sound recommendations when they emphasize that it is often necessary to take down the splenic flexure to achieve this goal. Taking down the splenic flexure routinely is also a means of guaranteeing a tension-free anastomosis.

According to these[2] and other recommendations[1,3,5], the upper or proximal limit should remove all proximal foci of inflammation, leading to a safe anastomosis. This implies sometimes performing a left colectomy.

The distal limit of excision, however, has given rise to much more discussion. Benn et al.[4], from the same Mayo Clinic in 1986; Mann, Goligher, and Hughes, in their respective textbook chapters, as well as more modern authors including Wexner et al.[8], Frizelle et al.[9], and Bergamaschi et al.[8,10] all advocated including the sigmoid rectal junction in the resection. Effectively, Benn and co-workers[4] published the outcome of 501 consecutive patients who had resection and anastomosis for diverticular disease at the Mayo Clinic between 1970 and 1975, with a median 45-month follow-up. Recurrent diverticulitis developed in 12.5% of patients undergoing colosigmoidostomy compared with 6.7% of those with colorectostomy ($p = 0.03$). Reoperation was required in 3.4% of the patients in whom the sigmoid colon was used as the distal anastomotic site, and in 2.2% of those in whom the rectum had been used ($p > 0.05$). No increase in the prevalence of anastomotic leaks or other perioperative complications were found in patients in whom the rectum had been mobilized and used for the anastomosis. The reoperation rate was higher (29%) for the former group compared to the group of patients with colorectostomy, but this difference was not found to be statistically significant. These authors concluded that the entire distal sigmoid colon should be removed during resection for diverticular disease and anastomosed to the upper rectum to avoid recurrent diverticulitis. Mann, Goligher, and others have all stated that the rates of recurrence and reoperations were higher when this was not the case, and that the rectum itself was rarely involved in diverticular disease. In order to anastomose the proximal colon to the upper rectum, these authors implied posterior mobilization of the rectum, removing no more than the intraperitoneal segment of the upper rectum. The junction is classically determined by the disappearance of the taenia coli and, alternatively by a change in the aspect of the serosa. The presence of taenia coli in the resection margin was associated with a statistically significant higher recurrence rate in the study by the Cleveland Clinic[10]. Histological evidence of inflammatory involvement of the taenia coli, often associated with diverticular disease[11,12], might be another element in favour of resecting the upper portion of the rectum to be sure that the specimen contains the colonic junction where the taenia disappear. Some surgeons prefer to check the site of the junction endoscopically during the procedure (Wexner, personal communication).

Anastomosis of the colon to the upper rectum does not, however, mean wide mobilization of the rectum and anastomosis to the middle or lower rectum. There are many studies that have shown that infraperitoneal colorectostomy is associated with higher anastomotic leakage rates, and increased overall morbidity and mortality[13,14]. Bergamaschi and Arnaud[5] are among the very few authors who, while recommending that the anastomosis be between the colon and the upper rectum, caution against entering the Douglas pouch to do so.

In the emergency setting the rules should be the same, especially since one- or two-stage treatments should include resection of the infected segment of colon as part of source control, completed by at least that of the sigmoid colon for the remaining diverticula, as indicated above. The problems stem from the degree of inflammation and the severity of peritonitis, which in some instances can lead to difficult decisions as to the extent of resection performed in this sometimes alarming setting. Two fairly recent controlled randomized studies – one in Denmark[15] and another in France[16] – looked at the best way to manage generalized peritonitis complicating sigmoid diverticulitis. Both of these studies, however, were relatively small. While the first study by Kronberg[15], was a monoinstitutional study which involved 62 patients and 27 surgeons, over a 14-year period, without any scoring system of severity, subgroup analysis seemed to indicate that secondary resection was preferred in the case of Hinchey III but outcome was better with resection (although not statistically so) in Hinchey IV patients. The proportion of patients who never underwent definitive resection of their sigmoid colon, however, was high: 14 of 31 or 45%. Critical appraisal of this paper and the results of the second study[16] are in favour of primary resection. As in the Kronberg study[15], Zeitoun and colleagues[16] compared primary resection and suture with drainage and proximal colostomy followed by secondary resection, but in a multicentre setting, including 105 patients and 34 surgeons over a 7-year period, and used the Mannheim Peritonitis Index. Their main endpoint was postoperative peritonitis, which occurred less often after primary than after secondary resection. Early reoperation was performed less often following primary resection than after secondary resection (2/55 vs 9/48 ($p<0.02$), leading to a shorter median first hospital stay (15 vs 24 days) ($p<0.05$). The mortality rate, however, did not differ significantly (24% vs 19%) overall or according the the Hinchey classification (27% Hinchey III vs 19% Hinchey IV). The authors[16] recommended primary resection in the treatment of generalized peritonitis complicating sigmoid diverticulitis, therefore indicating that the same recommendations as to the extent of resection can be applied safely in the emergency setting, even in the case of Hinchey III and IV. Other studies are ongoing (Bergamaschi, personal communication).

In some instances complicated diverticular disease takes the form of pseudotumoral masses or adherences which may lead the surgeon to perform a radical, carcinological-based resection.

In case of perforation into other organs the resection may be extended to other segments of the intestinal tract, such as the small intestines or a portion of the bladder, or sometimes the vaginal dome. The edges of the resected bladder or vagina can usually be closed by simple surgical means.

The problem of bleeding diverticula leads us to another dimension and to two unresolved problems: (1) is the bleeding due to diverticular disease and, if so, (2) what is the exact site of the source of bleeding? If adequate diagnostic work-up has either reasonably identified the source of bleeding as originating from a particular segment of the colon bearing diverticula, and/or when other plausible causes have been eliminated, and when continuous and/or severe bleeding menaces the vital prognosis, most authors[17–20] are in favour of surgical resection of the involved segment. Others[21] would try selective intra-arterial infusion of vasopressin and endoscopic injection haemostasis but, even if the haemorrhage can be stopped by non-surgical means, elective surgery should be considered to prevent recurrence in the long term[1]. When surgery is performed, on-table lavage and endoscopy should be considered to help localize the bleeding[22]. However, exact localization is often impossible[1,23]. In these cases every effort should be made to avoid repeat operations with progressive 'sausage-cutting': subtotal colectomy with ileorectal anastomosis is indicated[1].

Wexner's[10] and Bergamaschi's[5] groups recently compared the extent of resection between laparoscopic and traditional sigmoid resection, and confirmed that laparoscopic resection was equally adequate as regards the length of the specimen and the level of anastomosis. Bergamaschi and Arnaud[5], on the other hand, found a significantly shorter difference in the length of the specimen (11 ± 0.2 vs 18 ± 0.4 cm, $p < 0.01$) and the presence of inflammation in the proximal resection margin (11/40 laparoscopic colectomies vs 2/35 colectomies, $p < 0.02$) when the colectomy was performed laparoscopically, emphasizing further the need, above all in laparoscopic colectomy, not to hesitate to take down the splenic flexure in these patients, especially when the surgeon is on the so-called 'learning curve'.

As concerns the extent of resection of the mesocolon, this leads us to consider the vascularization of the sigmoid colon. One non-randomized study[24], and at least one randomized trial[25], have looked at the value of preservation of the superior rectal artery to ensure the vascularization of the rectal stump. In the first, a non-randomized but prospective study, involving patients undergoing sigmoid resection in the treatment of complete rectal prolapse, data on 33 selected patients were collected[24]. After withdrawal of three patients who had neither resection nor anastomosis, 29 women and one man (median age 55, range 21–83 years) underwent laparoscopic sigmoid resection (LSR) with preservation of the superior rectal artery (SRA). Mortality was nil. There were no anastomotic-related complications in the 30-day postoperative period. The authors[24] concluded that sparing the SRA had a favourable impact on anastomotic leak rates.

In a randomized controlled study[25] of 163 patients undergoing left colectomy for complicated diverticular disease of the colon, patients were allotted to two groups: in group A (n = 86 patients) the integrity of the inferior mesenteric artery (IMA) was preserved by artery skeletization; in group B (n = 77) the IMA was divided at its origin. The authors found the surgical time was longer in group A. Radiological and clinical leakages were significantly higher in group B ($p = 0.02$, $p = 0.03$, respectively) while a significantly lower number of staple-ring disruptions was observed, evolving into clinical dehiscence, in group A. The authors concluded that preserving the natural blood supply to the rectum, and the ensuing use of a healthy well-nourished rectal stump, are essential in preventing leakage and promoting adequate healing of the colorectal anastomosis.

The overall implications are that: (a) the splenic flexure should be taken down routinely to ensure a safe, tensionless anastomosis; (b) in laparoscopic surgery, the upper limit of the proposed resection should be landmarked with a clip before starting the dissection in order to be sure the entire proximal sigmoid is resected in the specimen; (c) the sigmoid rectal junction must be identified and resected in all cases; and (d) the colorectal anastomosis has to be performed intracorporeally, whether through a traditional laparotomy or by laparoscopy.

References

1. Köhler L, Sauerland S, Neugebauer E, for the Scientific Committee of the European Association for Endoscopic Surgery (EAES). Diagnosis and treatment of diverticular disease. Results of a consensus development conference. Surg Endosc. 1999;13:430–6.
2. Judd ES. Surgical treatment of diverticulitis of the colon. Ind Med Surg. 1955;24:443–6.
3. Leigh JE, Judd ES, Waugh JM. Diverticulitis of the colon: recurrence after apparently adequate segmental resection. Am J Surg. 1962;103:51–4.
4. Benn PL, Wolff BG, Ilstrup DM. Level of anastomosis and recurrent colonic diverticulitis. Am J Surg. 1986;151:269–71.
5. Bergamaschi R, Arnaud JP. Anastomosis level and specimen length in surgery for uncomplicated diverticulitis of the sigmoid. Surg Endosc. 1998;12:1149–51.
6. Munson KD, Hensien MA, Jacob LN, Robinson AM, Liston WA. Diverticulitis. A comprehensive follow-up. Dis Colon Rectum. 1996;39:318–22.
7. Wolff BG, Ready RL, MacCarty RL, Dozois RR, Beart RW. Influence of sigmoid resection on progression of diverticular disease of the colon. Dis Colon Rectum. 1984;27:645–7.
8. Thaler K, Baig MK, Berho M et al. Determinants of recurrence after sigmoid resection for uncomplicated diverticulitis. Dis Colon Rectum. 2003;46:385–8.
9. Frizelle FA, Dominguez JM, Santoro GA. Management of post-operative recurrent diverticulitis: a review of the literature. J R Coll Surg Edinb. 1997;42:1–6.
10. Thaler K, Weiss EG, Nogueras JJ, Arnaud JP, Wexner SD, Bergamaschi R. Recurrence rates at minimum 5-year follow-up: laparoscopic versus open sigmoid resection for uncomplicated diverticulitis. Surg Laparosc Endosc Percutan Tech. 2003;13:325–7.
11. Simpson J, Scholefield JH, Spiller RC. Pathogenesis of colonic diverticula. Br J Surg. 2002; 89:546–54.
12. Whiteway J, Morson BC. Pathology of the ageing-diverticular disease. Clin Gastgroenterol. 1985;14:829–46.
13. Schrock TR, Deveney CW, Dunphy JE. Factors contributing to leakage of colonic anastomosis. Ann Surg. 1973;177:513–18.
14. Alberts JCJ, Parvaiz A, Moran BJ. Predicting risk and diminishing the consequences of anastomotic dehiscence following rectal resection. Colorect Dis. 2003;5:478.
15. Kronberg O. Treatment of perforated sigmoid diverticulitis: a prospective randomized trial. Br J Surg. 1993;80:505–7.
16. Zeitoun G, Laurent A, Rouffet F et al. The French Association for Surgical Research multicentre, randomized clinical trial of primary versus secondary sigmoid resection in generalized peritonitis complicating sigmoid diverticulitis. Br J Surg. 2000;87:1366–74.
17. Bokhari M, Vernava AM, Ure T, Longo WE. Diverticular hemorrhage in the elderly – is it well tolerated? Dis Colon Rectum. 1996;39:191–5.
18. Foutch PG. Diverticular bleeding: are nonsteroidal anti-inflammatory drugs risk factors for hemorrhage and can colonoscopy predict outcome for patients? Am J Gastroenterol. 1995; 90:1779–84.
19. McGuire HH. Bleeding colonic diverticula. A reappraisal of natural history and management. Ann Surg. 1994;220:653–6.
20. Parkes BM, Obeid FN, Sorensen VJ, Horst HM, Fath JJ. The management of massive lower gastrointestinal bleeding. Am Surg. 1993;59:676–8.

21. Ramirez FC, Johnson DA, Zierer ST, Walker GJ, Sanowski RA. Successful endoscopic hemostasis of bleeding colonic diverticula with epinephrine injection. Gastrointest Endosc. 1996;43:167–70.
22. Allen Mersh TG. Should primary anastomosis and on-table colonic lavage be standard treatment for left colon emergencies? Ann R Coll Surg Engl. 1993;75:195–8.
23. Forde KA. Colonoscopy in acute rectal bleeding. Gastrointest Endosc. 1981;27:219–20.
24. Bergamaschi R, Lovvik K, Marvik R. Preserving the superior rectal artery in laparoscopic sigmoid resection for complete rectal prolapse. Surg Laparosc Endosc Percutan Tech. 2003; 13:374–6.
25. Tocchi A, Mazzoni G, Fornasari V, Miccini M, Daddi G, Tagliacozzo S. Preservation of the inferior mesenteric artery in colorectal resection for complicated diverticular disease. Am J Surg. 2001;182:162–7.

18
Surgery for diverticular disease: pro laparoscopy

M. H. MÜLLER, M. E. KREIS and K. W. JAUCH

INTRODUCTION

Laparoscopic-assisted sigmoid colectomy for recurrent diverticulitis has become increasingly popular throughout recent years in a vast number of hospitals[1]. One of the main and most obvious advantages is the superior cosmetic results following a laparoscopic-assisted sigmoid colectomy. While many surgeons master the technical requirements in order to perform this operation, the net evidence to support this approach as advantageous for the patient compared to the open operation remains limited. Here, we aim to review the studies and evidence that provide the basis for the argument that the laparoscopic-assisted technique is superior to the conventional approach.

COMPLICATIONS

In a review of several studies comparing laparosopic with conventional colorectal resections, the rate of overall complications was 20% following laparoscopy and 30% in open surgery[2] (Table 1). However, this applies mainly to minor complications such as infections, e.g. wound infections[3]. The rates of anastomotic leaks and postoperative mortality were not different[4]. It needs to be considered, however, that a certain bias may occur in these studies as laparoscopy is predominantly performed by specialized, well-trained and experienced surgeons, while open colectomy may also be undertaken by less-specialized surgeons, or as an operation to train residents at teaching hospitals. Furthermore, younger patients who are naturally less prone to have complications may frequently opt for laparoscopy based on cosmetic considerations, which may lead to a bias towards fewer complications following laparoscopic-assisted colectomy.

Table 1 Complications following open and aparosopic-assisted sigmoid colectomy

	Total complication rate		
Trial	*Open*	*Laparoscopic*	*p*
Braga	63/133	39/136	0.002
Hewitt	0/8	0/9	0.957
Curet	5/18	6/25	0.779
Leung	6/17	5/17	0.714
Lacy	37/108	14/111	<0.001
Neudecker	0/16	0/14	0.949
Milsom	8/54	8/59	0.848
Stage	0/16	2/18	0.268
Schwenk	8/30	2/30	0.038
Overall complication rate:	30%	20%	

IMMUNE RESPONSE

The immune response secondary to the operative trauma may be quantified by the number of specific subpopulations of immune cells that are present following laparosopic or open sigmoid colectomy. Wichmann et al. found no difference between these two operation for T-helper cells on postoperative days 1–5, while the number of natural killer cells was reduced on postoperative days 1 and 5 following open surgery[5]. Furthermore, reduced levels of IL-6 and C-reactive protein were documented after laparosopic-assisted versus open sigmoid colectomy[6]. While these investigations argue for a less pronounced immune response following laparoscopic surgery, the clinical relevance of these observations remains to be determined, although we would assume *a priori* that a reduced postoperative immune response should be advantageous for the patients.

POSTOPERATIVE RECOVERY/HOSPITAL STAY/POSTOPERATIVE ILEUS

Most colorectal surgeons will agree with the general impression that patients recover more quickly following laparoscopic procedures compared to conventional surgery. This, however, is difficult to demonstrate by objective parameters. One of these is that patients apparently require less postoperative pain medication when laparoscopic colectomy is performed[7]. Another parameter is the well-documented observation that postoperative hospital stay is shortened following laparoscopic surgery[4,7–9]. In a recent study investigating postoperative colonic motility it was found that motility recovers earlier following laparoscopic surgery compared to the conventional operation, which was associated with a shortened hospital stay[8]. It is of note, however, that others have also shown that very brief hospital stays are feasible following

Table 2 Controversy in treatment costs following open or laparoscopic-assisted sigmoid colectomy (**A**: mean costs in US$; **B**: mean costs in Euro)

A	*Open sigmoid colectomy*	*Laparoscopic sigmoid colectomy*
Pharmacy	433	269
Laboratory	123	64
Nursing	1476	676
Operation	1022	1785
Hospital stay	6	3
Total costs	3655	3209

B	*Open sigmoid colectomy*	*Laparoscopic sigmoid colectomy*
Total costs of first admission	5375	6931
Operation	3298	4734
Anaesthesia	555	703
Recovery room	366	287
Instruments	249	982
Other costs	176	280
Total costs of care after discharge	1860	2548
Re-admission	296	725
Post-operative stay	992	1035
Outpatient care	572	788
Total cost excluding productivity loss	7235	9479
Productivity loss	2579	2181
Total cost	9814	11 660

Modified from Delaney et al. 2003[9] and Janson et al. 2004[13],

conventional surgery when so-called fast-track protocols are applied[10]. This suggests that some of the apparent advantages following laparoscopic-assisted sigmoid colectomy may be secondary to the expectations of the staff in charge of the postoperative care which, again, may result in an observer bias favouring the laparoscopic approach.

COSTS

Studies investigating treatment costs are generally influenced by the type of cost that is included. For example, different results are to be expected when only the costs in the hospitals are considered, compared to studies including the ensuing costs that result from varying time before the patient is back to work after surgery. Furthermore, costs differ when they are calculated by the insurance company or the hospital administrator. Comparing the laparoscopic operation with the corresponding open procedure demonstrated that the costs for the operation are higher secondary to the use of expensive materials and – in general – longer operation time[11]. However, this is counterbalanced by reduced costs, which is explained by patients' more rapid recovery following laparoscopy with reduced postoperative hospitalization time. In a German study Köhler and Eypasch calculated that laparoscopic-assisted sigmoid colectomy costs 13% less compared to conventional sigmoid colectomy[12]. A similar cost-saving effect due to laparoscopy was reported by Delaney et al. for the situation in North America (Table 2A)[9], while Janson et al. found higher costs for laparoscopy versus open surgery in the United Kingdom (Table 2B)[13].

SUMMARY

The available evidence suggests that laparoscopic sigmoid colectomy is possible at similar cost for the hospital, as higher costs for resources (OR time, materials) are counterbalanced by a shortened hospital stay. The rate of minor complications appears to be reduced following laparoscopy, which may be secondary to a different level of training of the surgeons who master this technique. In conclusion, laparoscopic sigmoid colectomy seems to be advantageous compared to the open operation in several aspects of minor importance. However, the open operation and laparoscopic-assisted colectomy are similar as regards costs, major complications and mortality, so that the open operation is still justified, particularly in departments where the knowledge to perform the laparoscopic operation is not available.

References

1. Barlehner E, Decker T, Anders S, Heukrodt B. Laparoscopic surgery of rectal carcinoma. Radical oncology and late results. Zentralbl Chir. 2001;126:302–6.
2. Abraham et al. Abraham NS, Young JM, Solomon MJ. Meta-analysis of short-term outcomes after laparoscopic resection for colorectal cancer. Br J Surg. 2004;91:1111–24.
3. Vignali A, Braga M, Zuliani W, Frasson M, Radaelli G, Di Carlo V. Laparoscopic colorectal surgery modifies risk factors for postoperative morbidity. Dis Colon Rectum. 2004;47:1686–93.
4. Anthuber M, Fuerst A, Elser F, Berger R, Jauch KW. Outcome of laparoscopic surgery for rectal cancer in 101 patients. Dis Colon Rectum. 2003;46:1047–53.
5. Wichmann MW, Huttl TP, Winter H et al. Immunological effects of laparoscopic vs open colorectal surgery: a prospective clinical study. Arch Surg. 2005;140:692–7.
6. Schwenk W, Jacobi C, Mansmann U, Bohm B, Mueller MH. Inflammatory response after laparoscopic and conventional colorectal resections – results of a prospective randomized trial.Langenbecks Arch Surg. 2000;385:2–9.
7. Clinical Outcome of Surgical Therapy Study Group. A comparison of laparoscopically assisted and open colectomy for colon cancer. N Engl J Med. 2004;350:2050–9.
8. Kasparek MS, Mueller MH, Glatzle J et al. Postoperative colonic motility in patients following laparoscopic-assisted and open sigmoid colectomy. J Gastrointest Surg. 2003;7: 1073–81.
9. Delaney CP, Kiran RP, Senagore AJ, Brady K, Fazio VW. Case-matched comparison of clinical and financial outcome after laparoscopic or open colorectal surgery. Ann Surg. 2003;238:67–72.

10. Hjort Jakobsen D, Sonne E, Basse L, Bisgaard T, Kehlet H. Convalescence after colonic resection with fast-track versus conventional care. Scand J Surg. 2004;93:24–8.
11. Chapman AE, Levitt MD, Hewett P, Woods R, Sheiner H, Maddern GJ. Laparoscopic-assisted resection of colorectal malignancies: a systematic review. Ann Surg. 2001;234:590–606.
12. Köhler L, Eypasch E. Costs of laparoscopic colon surgery: are they justifiable? Chir Gastroenterol. 2001;17:34–9.
13. Janson M, Bjorholt I, Carlsson et al. Randomized clinical trial of the costs of open and laparoscopic surgery for colonic cancer. Br J Surg. 2004;91:409–17.

Section VIII
Medical treatment

Chair: R.C. SPILLER and M. STARLINGER

19
Medical management of diverticular disease: the role of bulking agents

J. LINDSAY

INTRODUCTION

The role of fibre in the aetiology and treatment of diverticular disease has been recognized in the gastroenterology literature for at least 40 years. In 1971 Burkitt and Painter described diverticulosis as a dietary deficiency of Western civilization, like scurvy, that could be avoided with an adequate diet[1]. A survey of 224 gastroenterologists at the World Congress in the mid-1970s would suggest that this opinion was widely held, as 75% of those surveyed recognized the role of fibre in the prevention and treatment of diverticular disease. However this confidence is not supported by the published literature, with only five randomized controlled trials primarily assessing the role of fibre in diverticular disease, which have included less than 250 patients in total. This chapter will discuss the classification of fibre, the proposed mechanism for action of fibre supplementation, and then describe the evidence of its role in the prevention of diverticulosis, the treatment of symptomatic diverticular disease, and prevention of complications relating to diverticular disease.

BULKING AGENTS: NON-STARCH POLYSACCHARIDES

Bulking agents used in the treatment of diverticular disease, like dietary fibre, are complex carbohydrates, which are resistant to digestion. The original classification that divided them into insoluble and soluble fractions, dependent upon their solubility at a predefined pH, has been superseded by the term 'non-starch polysaccharides' (NSP). The rationale for this is to standardize the chemical quantification of these carbohydrates. NSP are divided into cellulose which is insoluble, and non-cellulose polysaccharides which have variable solubility. The latter groups include sterculia, arabinogalactans, glucans, mucilages such as ispaghula, pectins, fungal chitins, and inulin. The common bulking agents such as Mucofalk, Fybogel, Isogel and Regulan contain ispaghula where as Normacol is made up of sterculia and Celevac is cellulose.

Non-starch polysaccharides, whether ingested as part of the normal dietary fibre or as bulking agents, have several actions on the human digestive system. First, they reduce bile reabsorption and increase its loss in the faeces. They blunt blood glucose responses and NSP high in phytates affect nutrient absorption (particularly of divalent cations and trace elements). Irrespective of their solubility in a laboratory all NSP are fermented to some extent by the colonic microbiota, allowing the production of short-chain fatty acids such as butyrate and acetone. Several of the NSP are selectively fermented by individual commensal bacterial strains and as such may affect the composition of the intestinal flora – a prebiotic effect. For example, inulin has been shown to increase the concentration of both faecal and mucosal-adherent bifidobacteria in healthy subjects. Their final action, dependent on the non-fermented fraction, is to increase stool bulk, resulting in faster whole-gut transit, and reduced intraluminal colonic pressures. It is important to remember that the increased stool bulk will result both from bacterial fermentation of the non-starch polysaccharide with subsequent microbial expansion, and also from a lack of fermentation leading to increased stool water content. This increased stool water content results from the faster colonic transit with subsequent reduction in water reabsorption, as well as from the water-retaining capacity of the NSP. In the United Kingdom the average intake of NSP is 12 g/day, resulting in a stool weight of 100 g/day. The recommended UK daily intake is 18g/day, which would result in a 25% increase in stool bulk as there is a linear relationship between NSP intake and stool weight, with intakes in the range of 4–32 g/day.

THE ROLE OF DIETARY NSP/BULKING AGENTS IN DIVERTICULAR DISEASE

There is a wide spectrum of diverticular disease ranging from the presence of diverticulosis, the generation of symptoms, progression towards diverticulitis, and subsequent complications such as colonic haemorrhage, diverticular colitis, and abscess formation. The role of non-starch polysaccharide has been studied in many of these situations. However, the majority of published research predates the reclassification of NSP and therefore quotes values for total fibre.

The incidence of diverticular disease has increased over the course of the past five decades. Likewise there is considerable geographic and ethnic variability and an increasing incidence with age. Several authors have suggested that this epidemiological variation results from alterations in the non-starch polysaccharide content of the diet. There is no doubt that the great geographical differences in the incidence of diverticular disease between sub-Sahara and Africa and the United Kingdom are correlated with alterations in the non-starch polysaccharide content of the diet, stool weight and whole-gut transit. Thus, in a review of 1200 subjects, the average United Kingdom stool weight was 110 g/day with a whole-bowel transit of 80 h, compared to the average Ugandan stool weight of 450 g/day with a transit of 34 h[2]. Within the UK population the role of fibre in the development of diverticulosis has been assessed between 56 vegetarians (mean intake of 41.5 ± 12.6 g of fibre per day) and 264 non-vegetarians (21.4 ± 8.2 g of fibre per day). All subjects were asymptomatic, and agreed to a single-contrast barium enema. Thirty-three per cent of non-vegetarians were found to have diverticular disease compared to 12% of the vegetarian population ($p < 0.01$). These highly significant results persisted when stratified for age. In addition there were significant differences in the fibre intake of vegetarians with diverticular disease, compared to those without[3]. Likewise fibre plays a role in the development of diverticulosis in animal models; 1900 Wistar rats were fed nine differing dietary regimes, and sacrificed after 18 months. Forty-five per cent of rats in the lowest-fibre groups had colonic diverticulosis, compared to 9% within the high-fibre group ($p < 0.01$)[4].

Several groups have investigated the potential pathogenic mechanisms of the effect of fibre in the development of diverticulosis. A necropsy study that compared colonic collagen in 20 unaffected colons, and five colons with diverticulosis, did not demonstrate differences in the total collagen content[5]. However, there was a significant increase in the insolubility of colonic collagen with age, which was more marked in the patients with diverticular disease. The sigmoid colon solubility index was 5.4 (SD 1.7) in subjects less than 60 years old, 10.3 (2.5) in subjects greater than 60 years old and 17.1 (2.8) in subjects with diverticulosis; $p < 0.001$). Further studies have demonstrated that this represents increased collagen crosslinking and hence rigidity in patients with diverticular disease. These findings are supported by an animal model: Wistar rats fed a low-fibre (17 g non-starch polysaccharide per kilogram per day) for 18 months were compared to rats ingesting a high-fibre diet (133 g/kg per day). The high-fibre diet induced a 70% increase in weight of the colonic contents and significant enhancement of faecal short-chain fatty acid concentration. Diverticula were present in 42% of the low-fibre group compared to none of the high-fibre group. As in the necropsy study, total collagen was similar in the two groups, but the collagen was relatively less soluble in the rats fed a low-fibre diet, with higher collagen crosslinkage[6].

THE ROLE OF FIBRE IN THE PREVENTION OF SYMPTOMS

It is obviously difficult to perform a study that looks into the role of fibre in preventing otherwise asymptomatic patients with diverticulosis from developing symptoms. Aldoori et al. examined this question in their prospective dietary cohort study of 43 881 medical professionals in the United States of America aged between 40 and 75 years[7,8]. All were free of symptomatic diverticular disease at the start of the study in 1986. They completed biannual dietary surveys until 1992. In the last two questionnaires (1990 and 1992) patients reported whether they had developed symptomatic diverticular disease. The response rate was 96% in 1990 and 94% in 1992. During 160 825 years of follow-up 362 cases of symptomatic diverticular disease were reported. The medical records of 182 patients who reported new-onset symptomatic diverticular disease were examined with 95% concordance. There was an inverse relationship between the dietary intake of non-starch polysaccharide and the risk of symptoms (relative risk 0.58, CI 0.41–0.83; p = 0.01). This effect was most significant for insoluble fibre (relative risk 0.63, CI 0.44–0.91; p = 0.02) and cellulose (relative risk 0.52, CI 0.36–0.75; p = 0.02).

THE ROLE OF FIBRE IN THE TREATMENT OF SYMPTOMATIC DIVERTICULAR DISEASE

The epidemiological evidence of an inverse correlation between dietary NSP intake and diverticular disease has led to considerable interest in the role of supplementation as a therapeutic strategy. An initial open-label study of 40 patients with symptomatic diverticular disease proven on barium enema looked at the benefit of 24 g of bran supplementation for 6 months[9]. There was a significant increase in stool weight and a reduction in colonic transit with the bran supplementation. This was associated with a significant decrease in the intraluminal colonic pressure in 32 out of the 39 patients studied. In validated symptom questionnaires, 33 out of the 40 patients had a symptomatic response, with 60% of the total reporting symptom burden being abolished. A subsequent double-blind placebo-controlled trial of wheat crisp bread (0.6 g fibre per day) versus bran crisp bread (6.7 g fibre per day) was performed in 18 patients with symptomatic diverticular disease[10]. Subjects completed a standardized symptom scale at monthly intervals, documenting symptoms of dyspepsia, abdominal pain, and colonic dysfunction. There was a significant reduction in the total symptom score in patients taking the high-fibre diet (from 34.3 to 8.1) compared to the control diet (from 42.0 to 35.1) over the 3-month study period ($p < 0.002$). There was also a significant reduction in abdominal pain ($p < 0.02$), but no significant difference in dyspepsia or bowel dysfunction.

These positive results were followed by a double-blind placebo-controlled crossover trial between ispaghula (9.04 g fibre per day), bran (6.99 g fibre per day) and a placebo (2.34 g fibre per day). Patients took each therapy for 4 months, and underwent both a subjective assessment of symptoms and an objective 7-day stool collection. The active treatment with ispaghula or bran resulted in a significant increase in stool weight and reduction of symptoms of constipation; however, there was no benefit above placebo in terms of abdominal pain, colonic dysfunction or total symptom score[11]. This led the authors to conclude that the role of fibre in diverticular disease was to treat underlying constipation rather than relieve symptoms relating to the diverticula themselves[12]. In support of this theory, controlled trials of fibre supplementation versus lactulose have not shown that fibre has a significant benefit over a simple laxative.

THE ROLE OF FIBRE IN PREVENTION OF DIVERTICULAR COMPLICATIONS

As with the therapy of symptomatic diverticular disease, there is limited evidence of the role of fibre in the prevention of complications relating to diverticular disease. The most comprehensive study is a retrospective review of

72 patients admitted to an English hospital with their first presentation of radiologically documented symptomatic diverticular disease[13]. Patients with complications such as strictures or abscesses were excluded. Patients with an elevated white cell count or pyrexia which might suggest diverticulitis were also excluded. Sixteen of the remaining patients with symptomatic simple diverticular disease underwent surgery as a primary therapy; the remaining 56 were treated conservatively, with 43 receiving dietary advice on fibre supplementation, of whom 31 were found to have subsequently complied (mean fibre intake in these patients 25 g per day). This group represented the high-fibre diet group. The low-fibre group comprised 13 patients not given dietary fibre supplementation, and the 12 patients who did not comply with dietary advice. Medium follow-up was 54 months in the high-fibre diet, and 76 months in the low-fibre diet. Patients taking a high-fibre diet underwent significantly fewer surgical procedures than those on a low-fibre diet (6.5% compared to 32%). Likewise patients on a high-fibre diet were significantly less likely to experience symptoms (19% compared to 44% with the low-fibre diet). This retrospective evidence would certainly suggest the protective role of fibre, but unfortunately there are no prospective trials to confirm this. Likewise there is no evidence of a role of fibre supplementation in the prevention of diverticular bleeding.

Diverticular colitis is a common complication of the condition, which may be divided into three pathological entities dependent on the histological similarity to ulcerative colitis, Crohn's disease or mucosal prolapse. Although little is known about the aetiology of this condition, suggested mechanisms have included ischaemia, prolapse of redundant mucosa, alterations in colonic short-chain fatty acid concentrations, stasis with subsequent toxin exposure and changes in the colonic microbiota[14]. NSP are an attractive therapeutic strategy as they impact on many of these mechanisms: they decrease colonic transit time and hence stasis, they reduce intracolonic pressure, they increase short-chain fatty acid release and finally they may have a prebiotic effect. However, there are no controlled trials of NSP in diverticular colitis and only open-label data to support their use.

SUMMARY

Dietary supplementation with non-starch polysaccharide results in an increased stool bulk and a decreased transit time. This is a consequence of the non-fermented component increasing stool water content, and the fermented component increasing bacterial bulk. Non-starch polysaccharide also results in an increase in short-chain fatty acid release, and may have prebiotic effects. There is good evidence of a role of non-starch polysaccharide in the prevention of diverticulosis, and in the prevention of the onset of symptoms. There is one small controlled trial suggesting a benefit of fibre supplementation in the treatment of symptomatic disease, although a larger trial would suggest that this benefit relates to its effect on relieving constipation. Retrospective data suggest that there may be a role for fibre in preventing the complications of diverticular disease, but this would need to be confirmed in larger studies.

In conclusion, fibre supplementation is a common prescription for patients with diverticular disease, although the evidence supporting its therapeutic efficacy is lacking. Given its safety, it will remain the mainstay of therapy for simple diverticular disease in most hospital settings. Caution should be exercised in the elderly, in whom excessive fibre supplementation may increase satiety, and decrease total calorie intake, as well as preventing the absorption of micronutrients.

References

1. Painter NS, Burkitt DP. Diverticular disease of the colon: deficiency disease of Western civilisation. Br Med J. 1971;2:450–4.
2. Burkitt DP, Walker ARP, Painter NS. Effect of dietary fibre on stools and transit times and its role in the causation of disease. Lancet. 1972;2:1408–12.
3. Gear JS, Furdson P, Nolan DJ. Symptomless diverticular disease and intake of dietary fibre. Lancet. 1979;1:511–14.
4. Fisher N, Berry CS, Fearn T et al. Cereal dietary fibre consumption and diverticular disease: a lifespan study in rats. Am J Clin Nutr. 1985;42:788–804.
5. Wess L, Eastwood MA, Wess TJ et al. Cross-linking of collagen is increased in colonic diverticulosis. Gut. 1995;37:91–4.
6. Wess L, Eastwood MA, Edwards C et al. Collagen alteration in an animal model of colonic diverticulosis. Gut. 1996;38:701–6.
7. Aldoori WH, Giovannuci El, Rimm EB et al. A prospective study of diet and the risk of symptomatic diverticular disease in men. Am J Clin Nutr. 1994;60:757–64.
8. Aldoori WH, Giovannucci El, Rockett HR. A prospective study of dietary fibre types and symptomatic diverticular disease in men. J Nutr. 1998;128:714–19.
9. Brodribb AJM, Humphreys DM. Diverticular disease: three studies. Part II. Treatment with bran. Br Med J. 1976;1:428–30.
10. Brodribb AJM. Treatment of symptomatic diverticular disease with a high fibre diet. Lancet. 1977;1:664–6.
11. Ornstein MH, Littlewood ER, Mclean Baird I et al. Are fibre supplementations really necessary in diverticular disease of the colon? A controlled clinical trial. Br Med J. 1981; 282:1353–6.
12. Otte JJ, Larsen L, Andersen JR. Irritable bowel syndrome and symptomatic diverticular disease – different diseases? Am J Gastroenterol. 1986;81:529–31.
13. Leahy AL, Ellis RM, Quil DS et al. High fibre diet in symptomatic diverticular disease of the colon. Ann R Coll Surg Engl. 1985;67:173–4.
14. Rampton DS. Diverticular colitis: diagnosis and management. Colorect Dis. 2001;3:149–53.

20 Antibiotics in the treatment of diverticular disease of the colon

G. LATELLA

INTRODUCTION

Diverticular disease of the colon is very common in Western developed societies[1–4]. It is associated with ageing and reduced intake of dietary fibre. Its incidence increases with age, and while it is uncommon before the age of 40 years, it is estimated to occur in about one-third of all individuals over 45 years of age, and in two-thirds of all those over 85 years[5–7]. Different prevalence rates have been reported in various geographic areas and ethnic groups[8,9]. The high prevalence of diverticular disease in developed Western countries is in contrast with its rarity in many developing countries and in Japan. Geographic correlation and time trend analyses suggest that the condition is the result of low intake of dietary fibre[8,9], a hypothesis supported by experimental[10,11], epidemiological[12–16] and therapeutic studies[17–19]. Indeed, in a prospective cohort study on approximately 50 000 health professionals, a significant inverse correlation has been found between insoluble dietary fibre intake and the risk of subsequently developing symptomatic diverticular disease[15]. Although the fibre-deficiency hypothesis has been widely quoted, conflicting findings and criticisms still exist[20–24].

Diverticular disease has a broad range of clinical manifestations. The majority of patients with diverticula of the colon remain asymptomatic all their life; a condition commonly referred to as diverticulosis or asymptomatic diverticular disease. About 20% of individuals with colonic diverticula develop symptoms characterized mainly by abdominal pain or discomfort, abdominal distension, and disturbances of bowel habits (mainly diarrhoea), the condition termed symptomatic diverticular disease, which may be symptomatic uncomplicated, recurrent symptomatic or complicated disease[2,5,6]. Symptomatic diverticular disease includes either the form without inflammation of the colon or that with inflammation termed diverticulitis, the latter affecting an estimated 10–25% of patients with the diasease[2,5,25]. Diverticultis is further subdivided into the uncomplicated and complicated forms. It has been stressed that clinical diverticulitis always represents a microperforation, demonstrating that in acute diverticulitis the colonic mucosa is macroscopic and histologically normal, despite marked inflammation of the pericolic tissue[26]. Less than 5% of patients will develop major complications such as perforation with abscess, diffuse peritonitis or fistula, obstruction, and massive bleeding[2–5]. Bleeding from diverticula is not associated with underlying acute inflammation; rather, the presumed cause of this complication is erosion of a submucosal blood vessel by impacted stool at the neck of a diverticulum. No reliable indicators are as yet available to distinguish patients who will become symptomatic from those who will not. Furthermore, no data have emerged indicating signs and symptoms that might predict the severity of the disease.

There is a general consensus that conservative treatment is indicated in patients with a first attack of uncomplicated diverticulitis, since about 70% of patients treated for a first episode will recover and have no further problems[6]. Those with recurrent attacks have a 60% risk of developing complications. Conservative treatment of diverticular disease is aimed at relief of symptoms and prevention of major complications[5,6,25]. Medical treatment of the diverticular disease of the colon includes bulking agents, antibiotics, probiotics, aminosalicylates, and anticholinergic/spasmolitic agents[27–30]. This chapter focuses on the use of antibiotics in the treatment of diverticular disease of the colon.

ANTIBIOTIC TREATMENT OF DIVERTICULAR DISEASE

Antibiotics are commonly used in the treatment of diverticular disease, although clinical trials, comparing antibiotics with placebo or even comparing various antibiotics, are lacking[5,6,27–30]. Their use is based on the general conditions of the patient, clinical experience and the hypothesis of bacterial involvement (Gram-negative and anaerobic bacteria). No specific enteric pathogens are responsible either for the symptoms or complications of the disease. On the contrary, the intestinal microflora seems to play an important role in this regard. The choice of antibiotic to be used varies according to the various clinical scenarios of the diverticular disease of the colon (Figure 1).

Asymptomatic diverticular disease

No data are so far available in support of any therapeutic recommendations or routine follow-up in the large population of patients with asymptomatic diverticular disease, although it is reasonable to recommend a high-fibre diet, also considering the potential health benefits of fibres in general[28,31]. Antibiotics should not be prescribed in this condition.

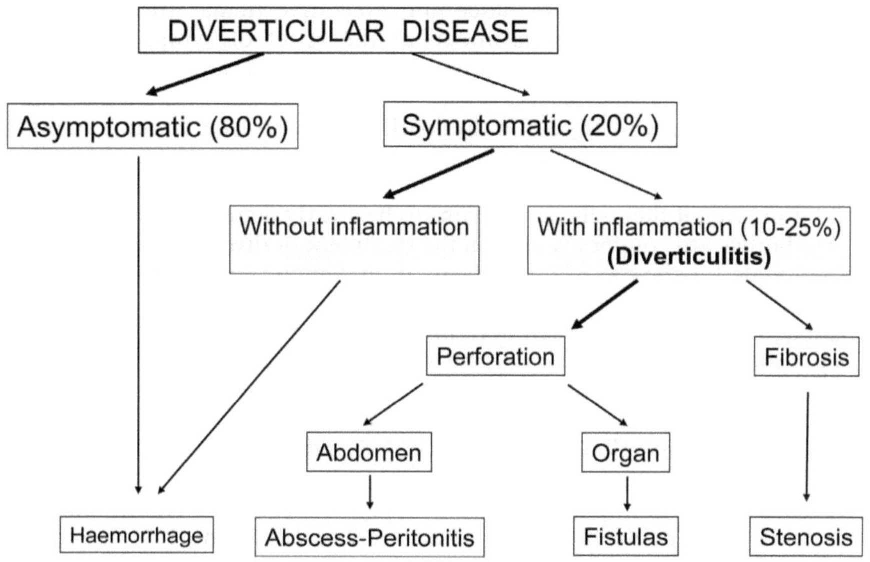

Figure 1 Flow chart indicating clinical scenarios of diverticular disease of the colon

Symptomatic uncomplicated diverticular disease without inflammation of the colon

Patients with this condition seek clinical attention for non-specific abdominal symptoms such as abdominal pain/discomfort, bloating, constipation, diarrhoea, passage of mucus, tenesmus, and abdominal tenderness. These patients are found to have diverticula of the colon without signs of colonic inflammation. Diverticulitis is usually excluded on the basis of clinical and laboratory signs (absence of rebound tenderness or other signs of peritoneal inflammation, and normal values of body temperature, leucocyte and erythrocyte sedimentation rate) with radiographic or endoscopic examinations (plain abdominal film, barium enema or colonoscopy, ultrasonography or CT scan, specifically performed on the basis of clinical findings) excluding any local inflammatory process of the colonic wall, perforation, abscesses or stenosis[6,28].

The relationship between these symptoms and the presence of colonic diverticula may be speculative. These non-specific symptoms overlap considerably with those of irritable bowel syndrome (IBS). It has even been postulated that colonic diverticula may be a late consequence of IBS[32,33]. Whether or not symptomatic uncomplicated diverticular disease without inflammation of the colon and IBS are distinct entities remains to be established, and is not clinically important, in as much as both are treated in a similar fashion, with equally good results.

Treatment of symptomatic uncomplicated diverticular disease without inflammation of the colon is aimed at the relief of symptoms and the prevention not only of the development of diverticulitis but also of major complications[6,28,31].

Although the efficacy of a high-fibre diet in the management of uncomplicated diverticular disease is still controversial, bran and bulking agents are commonly used. Likewise, antispasmodics are widely used in this condition, even if their efficacy remains to be clearly demonstrated.

Antibiotics are commonly used in the treatment of diverticulitis, but there is no rationale for the use of these agents in uncomplicated diverticular disease without inflammatory component[2–6,27–30,34,35]. However, data suggesting a possible role of intestinal microflora in determining some symptoms related to uncomplicated diverticular disease could be a rationale for the use of antibiotics in this subset of patients and, indeed, poorly absorbable antibiotics would probably be more suitable in this therapeutic purpose[36–41].

Constipation, as well as abdominal cramps and discomfort, are related to a reduction both of the intracolonic content and faecal bulk. The increase in faecal bulk with identical intake of dietary fibres seen after antimicrobial treatment is probably the result of an increased amount of non-degraded fibres in the faeces which, because of their water-holding capacity, bulks both the intracolonic content and the faeces[42]. Faecal bulking due to water-holding by undigested fibre would appear to be a more effective mechanism than the contribution by an increased bacterial mass. Non-degradable fibre seems to contribute to faecal bulking much more than an equal quantity of degradable fibre which bulks the faeces by increasing bacterial mass[43]. Non-fermentable fibre leads to an improvement in constipation and related abdominal pain, cramp and discomfort by increasing stool bulk, which stimulates peristalsis and reduces intracolonic pressure.

Intestinal bacterial fermentation of non-absorbed complex carbohydrates represents the major source of intestinal gas (H_2, CO_2, CH_4)[36]. Excessive production of bowel gas may play a role in determining abdominal symptoms such as bloating, pain and discomfort. Antibiotics have been shown to reduce colonic gas production and gas-related symptoms[37–40].

Bacterial overgrowth aided by faecal stasis inside the diverticula may be responsible for diarrhoea in diverticular disease[44–46]. Intestinal bacterial overgrowth-related diarrhoea is usually brought under control with antibiotics.

Therefore, a role of antibiotics in symptomatic uncomplicated diverticular disease without colonic inflammation may be suggested, with respect to their effects on fibre degradation, gas production, and bacterial overgrowth.

Of the poorly absorbable antibiotics currently available, the early aminoglycosides (neomycin, paramomycin) and the more recent rifamycin derivatives (rifaximin) are commonly used in the treatment of symptomatic uncomplicated diverticular disease (Figure 2).

There is evidence that long-term cyclic administration of poorly absorbed oral antibiotics, in particular rifaximin, leads to an improvement in symptoms in uncomplicated diverticular disease[31,47–49]. Rifaximin is a derivative of rifamycin with broad-spectrum bactericidal activity, including anaerobes[50,51]. It is virtually unabsorbed following oral administration.

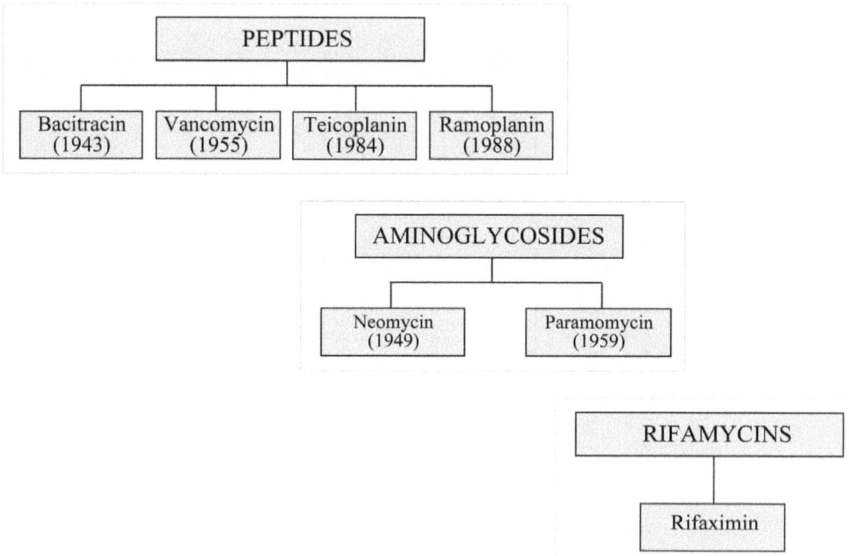

Figure 2 Poorly absorbed antibiotics currently used in the treatment of gastrointestinal infections, including diverticular disease of the colon. Modified from ref. 51

Open-labelled and randomized controlled trial data have shown that 1-year cyclic administration of rifaximin, combined with fibre supplementation, is safe and effective in obtaining symptom relief in uncomplicated diverticular disease of the colon[31,47–49] (Table 1). After 12 months the group of patients treated with rifaximin associated with fibre supplementation showed a significant reduction both in symptom occurrence rate (abdominal pain/discomfort, bloating, tenesmus, diarrhoea, abdominal tenderness) and in global symptomatic score, compared to the group treated with fibre alone. Overall, about 60% of the patients treated with rifaximin plus fibre and 30% of those treated with fibre alone were asymptomatic at 12 months. The advantage of the cyclic administration of rifaximin was proven by a significant reduction in the global symptomatic score after 4, 8 and 12 months, as compared to results of treatment with fibre alone (Figure 3) and by the percentage of asymptomatic patients (global symptomatic score = 0) after 12 months of treatment (approximately 60% vs 30%, respectively). This indicates a 30% therapeutic gain for rifaximin treatment as compared to fibre supplementation only. Considering the safety and tolerability of rifaximin, this agent could be usefully employed in the treatment of patients with symptomatic uncomplicated diverticular disease without colonic inflammation.

It is important to recall that symptoms attributed to colonic diverticula, such as pain or discomfort, bloating and bowel habits disorders (constipation or diarrhoea), are non-specific symptoms and are also features of irritable bowel

Table 1 Studies evaluating rifaximin in the treatment of symptomatic uncomplicated diverticular disease of the colon (data from refs 47–49)

Author (Study Design)	*Patients*	*Treatment*	*Study period (months)*	*Asymptomatic patients (%)*	*RD, % (95% CI)*	*Complications (%)*	*RD, % (95% CI)*
Papi 1992[47] (Open)	217	Glucomannan 2 g vs Glucomannan 2 g + rifaximin*	12	24 58	34.3 (22.0–46.5)	2.7 0.9	–1.8 (–5.3 to 1.7)
Papi 1995[48] (RCT)	168	Glucomannan 2 g + placebo vs Glucomannan 2 g + rifaximin*	12	39 69	29.7 (15.3–44.1)	2.3 2.3	0 (–4.6 to 4.6)
Latella 2003[49] (Open)	968	Glucomannan 4 g vs Glucomannan 4 g + rifaximin*	12	29 56	27.0 (20.9–33.1)	3.2 1.3	–1.8 (–3.8 to 0.1)

*Rifaximin 400 mg twice a day for 7 days each month for 12 months.

RD, rate difference ; 95% CI: 95% confidence interval; RCT, randomized controlled trial.

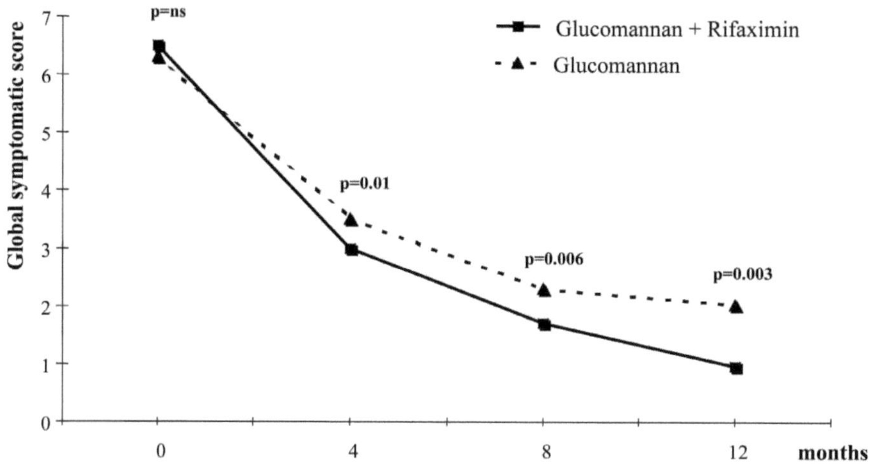

Figure 3 Global symptomatic score at baseline and at 4, 8 and 12 months of follow-up, according to the intention-to-tret analysis. Modified from ref. 49

syndrome (IBS). Also in IBS, intestinal microflora seems to play an important role in the development of such symptoms[41]. The hypothesis that diverticular disease and IBS may coexist, or even represent different phases of the same clinical condition, is also supported by the observation that, in many cases, these patients show either similar colon motility pattern or rectal pain sensation abnormalities[32,33]. Indeed, it has been reported that various antibiotics lead to a significant improvement in symptoms in IBS patients[52–54]; even constipation seems to show an improvement following antibiotics[55,56].

Therefore, the therapeutic effect of antibiotics, and in particular of the poorly absorbed antibiotics, is probably related primarily to colonic symptoms (or to colonic microflora) rather than to diverticula *per se*[31]. To unravel this aspect, future controlled clinical trials should include an additional arm of patients with IBS symptoms but not presenting colonic diverticula.

Another unsolved issue concerns the effectiveness of poorly absorbed antibiotics used in symptomatic uncomplicated diverticular disease in the prevention of diverticulitis and related major complications. As far as concerns the above-mentioned rifaximin trials, in two studies the incidence of diverticulitis or complications was lower in the group of patients treated with rifaximin plus fibre than in the group treated with fibre alone, while in the third study no differences were observed[47–49] (Table 1). However, in these studies the number of patients with diverticular disease complications during the 1-year follow-up period was too small to detect statistically significant differences between the two treatment groups. In a retrospective study on 505 patients admitted to hospital for diverticular disease complications and discharged after conservative treatment, long-term therapy with poorly absorbable antibiotics (neomycin, bacitracin, paramomycin, or rifaximin) reduced by 50% the relative risk of readmission for complications compared to no antibiotic treatment[57]. In addition, there is evidence that either rifaximin plus mesalazine or rifaximin plus probiotics seems to be effective in preventing diverticular disease complications[58–60].

No definitive conclusions can be drawn regarding a possible role of poorly absorbable antibiotics in preventing the development of diverticulitis and major complications of diverticular disease. Double-blind placebo-controlled trials are needed, but such trials are not easy to perform since a large number of patients are required. It has been estimated that a randomized controlled trial able to detect a 50% risk reduction in complications (assuming a baseline risk of diverticular disease complications of 5% per year)[2,5,6], should include at least 1600 patients per treatment group considering a study power of 80% ($1-\beta$) and an α error of 5%[31].

Symptomatic uncomplicated diverticular disease with inflammation of the colon (uncomplicated diverticulitis)

Diverticulitis results from inflammation and/or infection and subsequent perforation of colonic diverticula. It has been hypothesized that inflammation/infection of a diverticulum may develop when the diverticulum becomes obstructed by solid stool in its neck, subsequently leading to a perforation of the diverticula wall. The extent and localization of the perforation determines the clinical behaviour of colonic diverticula. Uncomplicated diverticulitis refers to diverticulitis with peridiverticulitis or phlegmon. Complicated diverticulitis refers to diverticulitis associated with abscess, free perforation, fistula, or obstruction[28,61].

Antibiotics are commonly used in the treatment of diverticulitis[5,6,25,27–30,61–65]. Variations in the management of uncomplicated diverticulitis have been reported, especially in terms of antibiotic choice, discharge instructions and follow-up of patients[35]. The choice of antibiotic should be based on the knowledge that Gram-negative rods and anaerobes are the usual bacteria involved in local infection[63,64]. Anaerobes are present, usually *Bacteroides fragilis*, in 65–90% of patients with intra-abdominal infections[66–68]. The decision as to whether or not to proceed with outpatient or inpatient treatment of the diverticulitis depends on the clinical judgement of the physician, severity of the disease, and likelihood that the patient's condition will respond to outpatient treatment.

Patients with mild diverticulitis can be treated as outpatients with a liquid diet and broad-spectrum oral antibiotics (nitroimidazoles, fluoroquinolones)[5,6,28–30,61] (Table 2). Patients with severe diverticulitis require hospitalization, bowel rest, intravenous fluid treatment and intravenous antibiotics active against the colonic anaerobic and Gram-negative flora, especially *Escherichia coli* and *Bacteroides*[5,6,28–30,61–65] (Table 3). Recommended antibiotic regimens, based more on clinical consensus than randomized controlled trials, include either the combination antibiotic regimens or single-agent coverage[64,65]. The former includes anti-anaerobic coverage with nitroimidazoles (e.g. metronidazole) or lincosamides (e.g.

Table 2 Antibiotic treatment of mild diverticulitis

Outpatient
Liquid diet
Oral antibiotics
Fluoroquinolones (e.g. ciprofloxacin)
+
Nitroimidazoles (e.g. metronidazole)

Table 3 Antibiotic treatment of severe diverticulitis

Hospitalization
Bowel rest
Intravenous antibiotics
Combined treatment
Nitroimidazoles (e.g. metronidazole) or lincosamides (e.g. clindamycin)
+
Aminoglycoside (e.g. gentamycin, tobramycin) or monobactam (aztreonam) or third-generation cephalosporin (ceftazidime, cefotaxime)
Single-agent treatment
Second-generation cephalosporin
cefoxitin, cefotetan
β4-lactamase inhibitors
ampicillin sodium/sulbactam sodium
piperacillin sodium/tazobactam sodium
ticarcillin disodium/clavulanate potassium
Carbapenems
imipenem–cilastin, meropenem
(Surgery)

clindamycin) and Gram-negative coverage with an aminoglycoside (e.g. gentamycin, tobramycin), monobactam (e.g. aztreonam) or third-generation cephalosporins (e.g. ceftazidime, cefotaxime). The latter approach offers a single-agent coverage with second-generation cephalosporins (e.g. cefoxitin, cefotetan) or β-lactamase inhibitor combinations (e.g. sulbactam–ampicillin, tircacillin–clavulanic acid, tazobactam–piperacillin) or carbapenems (e.g. imipenem–cilastatin, meropenem).

After recovery from the acute episode of diverticultis, a high-fibre diet is recommended. Long-term fibre supplementation after the first episode of diverticulitis may prevent recurrence in 70% of patients[69–71]. No data are yet available concerning the efficacy of long-term cyclic administration of poorly absorbed oral antibiotics in the prevention of diverticulitis recurrence and major complications.

Lack of improvement of diverticulitis with intensive conservative medical therapy suggests the need to search for complications of the disease, take into consideration an alternative diagnosis and have a surgical consultation. Surgery is recommended in patients with recurrent attacks of diverticulitis, patients with complicated disease, as well as in young or immunocompromised patients[5,6,28–30,61]. Diverticulitis is uncommon in young patients (<40 years old), but has a male predominance and is more virulent (higher rate of complications and need for surgery) than in the adult/elderly patients[72–76]. Immunocompromised patients had a higher rate of free perforation, need for surgery and postoperative mortality than the non-compromised patients[77–79].

Since diverticulitis recurs in a small percentage of patients, surgery is not generally indicated after a single uncomplicated episode of diverticulits[5,6,28–30,61]. Intravenous antibiotics are always recommended in the perioperative period of any surgical procedure performed for diverticular disease of the colon.

Complicated diverticular disease

The most frequent complications of diverticular disease are those related to acute diverticulitis including perforation with abscess, diffuse peritonitis, fistula, and obstruction[2–6,28,61]. Massive bleeding is much more commonly associated with colonic diverticula without colonic inflammation than with diverticulitis.

A grading system has been described reflecting the degree of perforation[70]: Stage I, diverticulitis associated with pericolic abscess; Stage II, diverticulitis associated with distant abscess (retroperitoneal or pelvic); Stage III, diverticulitis associated with purulent peritonitis; Stage IV, diverticulitis associated with faecal peritonitis.

Treatment of diverticular abscesses depends on their size, complexity and location, as well as on the patient's clinical condition at the time of diagnosis. Patients always require hospitalization, bowel rest, intravenous fluid treatment and intravenous antibiotics (combination of antibiotics or single antibiotic). Small pericolic abscesses (Stage I) may respond successfully to antibiotic therapy and bowel rest[28,61,80]. In those cases in which surgery is necessary, a single-stage resection and reanastomosis can be performed. Distant and large abscesses (Stage II) require prompt antibiotic treatment associated with percutaneous or surgical drainage. The advantage of percutaneous drainage is that it may lead to stabilization of the patient and then allow a single-stage resection and reanastomosis[28,61,81–83]. Drainage of abscesses at laparoscopy may be a useful procedure if CT scan- or ultrasound-guided drainage are unsuccessful, unavailable or contraindicated. Pyogenic liver abscesses may complicate colonic diverticulitis and they may require not only antibiotics but also percutaneous drainage[28]. Diverticulitis associated with free perforation (Stage III and IV) requires intensive medical treatment with total parenteral nutrition, antibiotics, cardiovascular and respiratory support, as well as emergency surgery; the procedure of choice in this situation is immediate segmental resection with colostomy[61].

When a diverticular phlegmon or abscess extends or leaks into an adjacent organ, fistulas may occur. Colovesical fistulas are the most common, comprising about 65% of diverticular fistulas[61]. Other fistulas include colovaginal, colocutaneous, coloenteric, and colouterine. Surgical resection is usually carried out with fistula closure[28,61,84,85]; antibiotics alone are not effective.

Colonic obstruction may complicate diverticular disease, either acutely or chronically[28,61]. During an episode of acute diverticulitis a partial colonic obstruction may occur caused by luminal narrowing from the pericolic inflammation or the compression from abscess formation. Colonic ileus or acute pseudo-obstruction may also occur. These conditions of acute colonic obstruction usually respond to antibiotic treatment. The obstruction improves as the inflammation subsides. Recurrent attacks of diverticulitis can give rise to progressive segmental fibrosis and stricturing of the colon wall that may lead to high-grade or complete obstruction requiring surgical resection. Endoscopic procedures have also been proposed in the treatment of these colonic fibrotic strictures[86,87].

Severe bleeding has been reported to occur in 3–5% of all patients with colonic diverticula[88]. Bleeding ceases spontaneously in approximately 80% of cases, with a rebleeding rate of about 30%[89]. Data suggesting that non-steroidal anti-inflammatory drugs may be implicated in diverticular bleeding have been reported[90,91]. It is crucial to localize and treat the bleeding source. Diagnostic options include colonoscopy and angiography which may also be a useful therapeutic approach in patients with ongoing bleeding, proceeding with surgery only in those cases in which the haemorrhage is not brought under control[28].

In conclusion, as far as concerns the complications of diverticular disease, antibiotics are of primary importance in the treatment of abscesses and free perforations, whereas in cases of fistulas, stenosis and haemorrhage their role is limited to that of perioperative prophylaxis.

References

1. Parks TG. Natural history of diverticular disease of the colon. Clin Gastroenterol 1975;4: 53–69.
2. Almy TP, Howell DA. Diverticular disease of the colon. N Engl J Med. 1980;302:324–31.
3. Ozick LA, Salazar CO, Donelson SS. Pathogenesis, diagnosis, and treatment of diverticular dsease of the colon. Gastroenterologist. 1994;2:299–310.
4. Simpson J, Spiller R. Colonic diverticular disease. Clin Evid 2003;9:478–87.
5. Ferzoco LB, Raptopoulos V, Silen W. Acute diverticulitis. N Engl J Med. 1998;338:1521–6.
6. Kohler L, Sauerland S, Neugebauer E, for the Scientific Committee of the European Association for Endoscopic Surgery (EAES). Diagnosis and treatment of diverticular disease. Results of a consensus development conference. Surg Endosc. 1999;13:430–6.
7. Farrell RJ, Farrell JJ, Morrin MM. Diverticular disease in the elderly. Gastroenterol Clin N Am. 2001;30:475–496.
8. Painter NS, Burkitt DP. Diverticular disease of the colon: a deficiency disease of Western civilization. Br Med J. 1971;2:450–4.
9. Painter NS, Burkitt DP. Diverticular disease of the colon: a 20th Century problem. Clin Gastroenterol. 1974;4:3–21.
10. Hodgson WJB. An interim report on the production of colonic diverticula in the rabit. Gut. 1972;13:802–4.
11. Fisher N, Berry CS, Feam T et al. Cereal dietary fiber comsumption and diverticular disease: a lifespanm study in rats. Am J Clin Nutr. 1985;42:788–804.
12. Brodribb AJM, Humphreys DM. Diverticular disease: three studies. I. Relation to other disorders and fibre intake. Br Med J. 1976;1:424–30.
13. Gear JSS, Ware A, Fursdon P, et al. Symptomless diverticular disease and intake of dietary fiber. Lancet. 1979;1:511–14.
14. Manousos O, Day NE, Tzonou A et al. Diet and other factors in the aetiology of diverticulosis: an epidemiological study in Greece. Gut. 1985;26:544–9.

15. Aldoori WH, Giovannucci EL, Rimm EB et al. A prospective study of diet and the risk of symptomatic diverticular disease in men. Am J Clin Nutr. 1994;60:757–64.
16. Aldoori WH, Giovannucci EL, Rockett HRH et al. A prospective study of dietary fiber types and symptomatic diverticular disease in men. J Nutr. 1998;128:714–19.
17. Brodribb AJM. Treatment of symptomatic diverticular disease with high-fibre diet. Lancet. 1977:1:664–6.
18. Weinreich J. The treatment of diverticular disease. Scand J Gastroenterol. 1982;79(Suppl.): 128–9.
19. Ewerth S, Ahlberg J. Holmstrom B. et al. Influence on symptoms and transit time of Vi Siblin R in diverticular disease. Acta Chir Scand (Suppl.). 1990;500:40–59.
20. Davey WW. Diet and diverticulosis. Br Med J. 1968;1:118–20.
21. Archampong EQ, Christian F, Badoe EA. Diverticular disease in an indigenous African community. Ann R Coll Surg Engl. 1978;60:464–70.
22. Ornestein MH, Littlewood ER, Baird IM, et al. Are fibre supplements really necessary in diverticular disease of the colon? A controlled clinical trial. Br Med J. 1981;282:1353–6.
23. Hodgson WJB. The placebo effect: is it important in diverticular disease? Am J Gastroenterol. 1977;67:157–62.
24. Mendeloff AI. A critique of 'fibre deficiency'. Am J Dig Dis. 1976;21:109–12.
25. Thompson DA, Bailey HR. Management of acute diverticulitis with abscess. Sem Colon Rectal Surg. 1990;1:74–80.
26. Fleischner FG, Ming SC. Revised concepts on diverticular disease of the colon. II. So-called diverticultis: diverticular sigmoiditis and perisigmoiditis, diverticular abscess, fistula, and frank peritonitis. Radiology. 1965;84:599–609.
27. Cheskin LJ, Lamport RD. Diverticular disease. Epidemiology and pharmacological treatment. Drugs Aging. 1995;6:55–63.
28. Stollmann NH, Raskin JB. Diagnosis and management of diverticular disease of the colon in adults. Am J Gastroenterol. 1999;94:3110–21
29. Tursi A. Acute diverticulitis of the colon – current medical therapeutic management. Expert Opin Pharmacother. 2004;5:55–9.
30. Buchanan GN, Kenefick NJ, Cohen CR. Diverticulitis. Best Pract Res Clin Gastroenterol. 2002;16:635–47.
31. Papi C, Koch M, Capurso L. Management of diverticular disease: is there room for rifaximin? Chemotherapy. 2005;51(Suppl. 1):110–14.
32. Ritchie J. Similarity of bowel distension characteristics in the irritable bowel syndrome and diverticulosis. Gut. 1977;18:A990.
33. Otte JJ, Larsen L, Anderson JR. Irritable bowel syndrome and symptomatic diverticular disease – different diseases? Am J Gastroenterol. 1986;81:529–31.
34. Torsoli A, Inoue M, Manousos O et al. Diverticular disease of the colon. Data relevant to treatment. Gastroenterol Int. 1991;4:3–20.
35. Schechter S, Mulvey J, Eisenstat TE. Management of uncomplicated acute diverticulitis. Results of a survey. Dis Colon Rectum. 1999;42:470–6.
36. Strocchi A, Levitt MD. Intestinal gas. In: Sleisenger MH, Fordtran JS, editors. Gastrointestinal Disease: Pathophysiology, Diagnosis, Management, 5th edn. Philadelphia: Saunders, 1993:1035–42.
37. Bjorneklett A, Midvedt T. Influence of three antimicrobial agents – penicillin, metronidazole and doxycyclin – on the intestinal microflora of healthy humans. Scand J Gastroenterol. 1988;94:928–32.
38. Rao SC, Edwards CA, Austen CJ, Bruce C, Read NW. Impaired colonic fermentation of carbohydrate after ampicillin. Gastroenterology. 1988;94:928–32.
39. Di Stefano M, Strocchi A, Malserviti S, Veneto G, Ferrieri A, Corazza GR. Non-absorbable antibiotics for managing intestnal gas production and gas-related symptoms. Aliment Pharmacol Ther. 2000;14:1001–8.
40. Di Stefano M, Malservisi S, Veneto G, Ferrieri A, Corazza GR. Rifaximin versus chlortetracycline in the short term treatment of small intestine bacterial overgrowth. Aliment Pharmacol Ther. 2000;14:551–6.
41. Lin HC. Small intestinal bacterial overgrowth: a framework for understanding irritable bowel syndrome. J Am Med Assoc. 2004;292:852–8.
42. Kurpad AV, Shetty PS. Effects of antimicrobial therapy on faecal bulking. Gut. 1986;27:55–8.

43. Stephen AM, Cummings IH. Mechanisms of action of dietary fibre in the human colon. Nature. 1980;284:183–4.
44. Toskes PP, Donalson RM. Enteric bacterial flora and bacterial overgrowth syndrome. In: Sleisenger MH, Fordtran TS, editors, Gastrointestinal Disease: Pathophysiology, Diagnosis, Management, 5th edn. Philadelphia: Saunders, 1993:1106–17.
45. Husebye E. The pathogenesis of gastrointestinal bacterial overgrowth. Chemotherapy. 2005;51(Suppl. 1):1–22.
46. Tursi A, Brandimarte G, Giorgetti GM, Elisei W. Assessment of small intestinal bacterial overgrowth in uncomplicated acute diverticulitis of the colon. World J Gastroenterol. 2005; 11:2773–6.
47. Papi C, Ciaco A, Koch M, Capurso L and Diverticular Disease Study Group. Efficacy of rifaximin on symptoms of uncomplicated diverticular disease of the colon. A pilot multicentre open trial. Ital J Gastroenterol. 1992;24:452–6.
48. Papi C, Ciaco A, Koch M, Capurso L. Efficacy of rifaximin in the treatment of symptomatic diverticular disease of the colon. A multicentre double-blind placebo-controlled trial. Aliment Pharmacol Ther. 1995;9:33–9.
49. Latella G, Pimpo MT, Sottili S et al. Rifaximin improves symptoms of acquired uncomplicated diverticular disease of the colon. Int J Colorectal Dis. 2003;18:55–62.
50. Gillis JC, Brogden RN. Rifaximin. A review of its antibacterial activity, pharmacokinetic properties and therapeutic potential in conditions mediated by gastrointestinal bacteria. Drugs. 1995;49:467–84.
51. Scarpignato C, Pelosini I. Rifaximin, a poorly absorbed antibiotic: pharmacology and clinical potential. Chemotherapy. 2005;51(Suppl. 1):36–66.
52. Nayak AK, Kamad DR, Abraham P, Mistry FP. Metronidazole relieves symptoms in irritable bowel syndrome: the confusion with socalled 'chronic amebiasis'. Indian J Gastroenterol. 1997;16:137–9.
53. Pimentel M, Chow EJ, Lin HC. Normalization of lactulose breath testing correlates with symptom improvement in irritable bowel syndrome. A double-blind, randomized, placebo-controlled study. Am J Gastroenterol. 2003;98:412–19.
54. Madden JA, Hunter JO. A review of the role of the gut microflora in irritable bowel syndrome and the effect of probiotics. Br J Nutr. 2002;88(Suppl. 19:S67–72.
55. Celik AF, Tomlin J, Read NW. The effects of oral vancomycin on chronic idiopathic constipation. Aliment Pharmacol Ther. 1995;9:63–8.
56. Bernay P, Houver A, Carraz M, Castel G. Study of fecal flora in constipated patients. Their modification by treatment with rovamycin–diphetarsone. J Med Lyon. 1967;48:847–54.
57. Porta E, Germano A, Ferrieri A, Koch M. The natural history of diverticular disease of the colon: a role for antibiotics in preventing complications? A retrospective study. Eur Rev Med Pharmacol Sci. 1994;16:33–9.
58. Tursi A. Preventive therapy for complicated diverticular disease of the colon; looking for a correct therapeutic approach. Gastroenterology. 2004;127:1865–6.
59. Fric P, Zavoral M. The effect of non-pathogenic *Escherichia coli* in symptomatic uncomplicated diverticular disease of the colon. Eur J Gastroenterol Hepatol. 2003;15: 313–15.
60. Tursi A. Mesalazine for diverticular disease of the colon – a new role for an old drugs. Expert Opin Pharmacother. 2005;6:69–74.
61. The standards task force of the American Society of Colon and Rectum Surgeon. Practice parameters for sigmoid diverticulitis – supporting documentation. Dis Colon Rectum. 1995;38:126–32.
62. Ertan A. Colonic diverticulitis: recognizing and managing its presentations and complications. Postgrad Med. 1990;88:67–72.
63. Duma RJ, Kellum JM. Colonic diverticulitis: microbiologic, diagnostic and therapeutic considerations. Curr Clin Top Infect Dis. 1991;11:218–47.
64. Kellum JM, Sugerman HJ, Coppa GF et al. Randomized prospective comparison of cefoxitin and gentamycin–clindamycin in the treatment of acute colon diverticulitis. Clin Ther. 1992;14:376–84.
65. Drusano GL, Warren JW, Saah AJ et al. A prospective randomized controlled trial of cefoxitin versus clindamycin–aminoglycoside in mixed anaerobic–aerobic infections. Surg Gynecol Obstet. 1982;154:715–20.
66. Nichols RL. Management of intra-abdominal sepsis. Am J Med. 1986;80:204–9.

67. Elsakr R, Johnson DA, Younes Z, Oldfield EC. Antimicrobial treatment of intra-abdominal infections. Dig Dis. 1998;16:47–60.
68. Younez Z, Johnson DA. New developments and concepts in antimicrobial therapy for intra-abdominal infections. Curr Gastroenterol Rep. 2000;2:277–82.
69. Larson DM, Masters SS, Spiro HM. Medical and surgical therapy in diverticular disease: a comparative study. Gastroenterology. 1976;71:734–7.
70. Hinchey EF, Schaal PG, Richards GK. Treatment of perforated diverticular disease of the colon. Adv Surg. 1978;12:85–109.
71. Painter NS. Diverticular disease of the colon: the first of the Western diseases shown to be due to a deficiency of dietary fiber. S Afr Med J. 1982;61:1016–20.
72. Freischlang J, Bennion RS, Thompson JE. Complications of diverticular disease of the colon in young people. Dis Colon Rectum. 1986;29:639–43.
73. Acosta JA, Grebenc ML, Doberneck RC et al. Colonic diverticular disease in patients 40 years old or younger. Am Surg. 1992;58:605–7.
74. Konvolinka CW. Acute diverticulitis under age forty. Am J Surg. 1994;167:562–5.
75. Vignati PV, Welch JP, Cohen JL. Long-term management of diverticulitis in young patients. Dis Colon Rectum. 1995;38:627–9.
76. Spivak H, Weinrauch S, Harvey JC, Surick B, Ferstenberg H, Friedman I. Acute colonic diverticulitis in the young. Dis Colon Rectum. 1997;40:570–4.
77. Perkins JD, Shield CF, Chang FC et al. Acute diverticulitis: comparison of treatment in immunocompromised and non-immunocompromised patients. Am J Surg. 1984;148:745–8.
78. Tyau ES, Prystowsky JB, Joehl RJ et al. Acute diverticulitis: a complicated problem in the immunocompromised patient. Arch Surg. 1991;126:855–9.
79. Schoetz DJ. Uncomplicated diverticulitis: indications for surgery and surgical management. Surg Clin N Am. 1993;73:965–74.
80. Ambrosetti P, Robert J, Witzing JA et al. Incidence, outcome, and proposed management of isolated abscesses complicating acute left-side colonic diverticulitis: a prospective study of 140 patients. Dis Colon Rectum. 1992;35:1072–6.
81. Stabile BE, Puccio E, Van Sonnemberg E et al. Preoperative percutaneous drainage of diverticular abscesses. Am J Surg. 1990;159:99–105.
82. Schecter S, Eisenstat TE, Oliver GC et al. Computed tomographic scan-guided drainage of intra-abdominal abscesses. Dis Colon Rectum. 1994;37:984–8.
83. Wedell J, Banzhaf G, Chaoui R et al. Surgical management of complicated colonic diverticulitis. Br J Surg. 1997;84:380–3.
84. Woods RJ, Lavery IC, Fazio VW, Jagelman DG, Weakley FL. Internal fistulas in diverticular disease. Dis Colon Rectum. 1988;31:591–6.
85. Pontari MA, McMillen MA, Garvey RH, Ballantyne GH. Diagnosis and treatment of enterovesical fistulae. Am Surg. 1992;58:258–63.
86. Kozarek RA. Hydrostatic balloon dilatation of gastrointestinal stenoses: a national survey. Gastrointest Endosc. 1986;32:15–19.
87. Oz MC, Forde KA. Endoscopic alternatives in the management of colonic strictures. Surgery. 1990;108:513–19.
88. Reinus JF, Brandt LJ. Vascular ectasias and diverticulosis: common causes of lower intestinal bleeding. Gastroenterol Clin N Am. 1994;23:1–20.
89. McGuire HH. Bleeding colonic diverticula: a reappraisal of natural history and management. Ann Surg. 1994;220:653–6.
90. Foutch PG. Diverticular bleeding: are nonsteroidal anti-inflammatory drugs risk factors for hemorrhage and can colonoscopy predict outcome for patients. Am J Gastroenterol. 1995; 90:1779–84.
91. Aldoori WH, Giovannucci EL, Rimm EB et al. Use of acetominophin and nonsteroidal anti-inflammatory drugs: a prospective study and the risk of symptomatic diverticular disease in men. Arch Fam Med. 1998;7:255–60.

21 Aminosalicylates

V. GROSS

INTRODUCTION

Aminosalicylates show a broad spectrum of anti-inflammatory activity. They inhibit many key factors of the inflammatory cascade, e.g. cyclo-oxygenase, thromboxan synthetase, platelet-activating factor synthetase, production of interleukin-1 and of free radicals. Aminosalicylates have an antioxidant activity. In addition, they interfere with the interaction of intestinal bacteria and epithelial cells. This may be the rationale for the use of aminosalicylates for the prevention and treatment of symptomatic diverticular disease. Symptomatic diverticular disease comprises a wide spectrum of pathological conditions ranging from slight mucosal irritation to perforated diverticulitis. In acute diverticulitis treatment with antibiotics is indispensable, but aminosalicylates could produce favourable effects in the long-term treatment and prevention of relapses. This question has therefore been addressed by several studies.

ANTI-INFLAMMATORY ACTIVITY OF AMINOSALICYLATES

Inflammation is triggered and maintained by many mediators which work in combination or may even have synergistic effects on each other. Investigations into the mechanism of action of 5-aminosalicylic acid have concentrated on the cells and mediators involved in the inflammatory reaction and on the epithelial cells of the mucosa and their barrier function.

5-Aminosalicylic acid has effects on prostaglandins and leukotrienes. While some studies showed an inhibition of prostaglandin synthesis[1,2], others showed an increase in prostaglandin production or a concentration-dependent effect[3,4]. In addition, aminosalicylates interfere with leukotriene production[5–7].

Oxidative stress plays an important role in tissue damage in inflammation. Phagocytic leucocytes which are found in large numbers in inflamed tissue are very probably the source of oxygen radicals. Aminosalicylates have antioxidant properties *in vitro* and can scavenge free radicals[8-10]. Ahnfelt-Rønne et al.[11] investigated metabolites of 5-aminosalicylic acid produced *in vitro* from oxygen radicals and *in vivo* in patients with inflammatory bowel disease receiving sulphasalazine, and postulated clinical relevance for the ability of 5-aminosalicylic acid to scavenge oxygen radicals.

Cytokines play an important role in inflammatory reactions. Mahida et al.[12] and Rachmilewitz et al.[13] demonstrated in colon biopsies from patients with chronic inflammatory bowel disease that 5-aminosalicylic acid is an inhibitor of interleukin-1 synthesis. Greenfield et al.[14] reported that the TNF-α induced increase in surface expression of specific adhesion molecules was inhibited by 5-aminosalicylic acid.

Platelet-activating factor (PAF) is also an important inflammatory mediator. In *in-vitro* investigations using rectal mucosal biopsy specimens from patients with ulcerative colitis and Crohn's disease, 5-aminosalicylic acid inhibited the stimulated secretion of PAF[15].

Various studies have shown that 5-aminosalicylic acid inhibits the chemotaxis of human neutrophils[16–18]. 5-Aminosalicylic acid also suppresses the stimulated histamine secretion from human intestinal mast cells and basophilic cells[19,20].

According to recent results 5-aminosalicylic acid seems to interfere with the interaction of intestinal bacteria and epithelial cells (Lochs et al., personal communication).

The broad spectrum of anti-inflammatory activity of aminosalicylates is the rationale for their use in symptomatic diverticular disease (Table 1).

Table 1 Anti-inflammatory activity of 5-ASA

Prostaglandin synthesis
Leukotriene synthesis
Thromboxane synthesis
PAF synthesis
Cytokines (IL-1, TNF)
Reactive oxygen metabolites

USE OF 5-AMINOSALICYLIC ACID IN DIVERTICULAR DISEASE

In acute diverticulitis treatment with antibiotics is indispensable, but aminosalicylates could have favourable effects in the long-term treatment and prevention of relapses. This question has been addressed by several studies.

Trespi et al.[21] evaluated the therapeutic and prophylactic role of 5-aminosalicylic acid in symptomatic diverticular disease of the colon. They performed a prospective study in 166 patients with mild to moderate symptomatic diverticular disease. The patients were initially treated with sulbactam/ampicillin 1.5 g i.m., and rifaximin 400 mg b.i.d. per os for 7 days. Following randomization the patients then received supplementary treatment with 5-aminosalicylic acid (400 mg b.i.d.) or no other treatment from weeks 2 to 9. Eighty-one patients received 5-aminosalicylic acid, 85 patients no supplementary treatment. After 4 years of follow-up, 44 patients had dropped out of the study (nine because of major complications, three because of massive haemorrhage and 32 for other reasons). Symptomatic recurrence of diverticular disease occurred in 12 patients treated with mesalazine and in 39 patients who had received no supplementary treatment (Figure 1). Minor diverticular haemorrhages occurred in 12 patients treated with mesalazine and in 31 patients who had received no supplementary treatment (Figure 2). The authors calculated a significantly increased probability of remaining free from symptomatic relapse ($p = 0.00005$) and from microhaemorrhagic phenomena ($p = 0.001$) for the mesalazine group. The duration of abdominal pain due to diverticulitis was also shorter in the group of patients treated with 5-aminosalicylic acid, while the incidence of major complications and of side-effects was comparable in the two groups. The authors concluded from these data that the supplementary short-time treatment with 5-aminosalicylic acid for 8 weeks had long-term (up to 48 months) beneficial effects in patients with symptomatic diverticular disease.

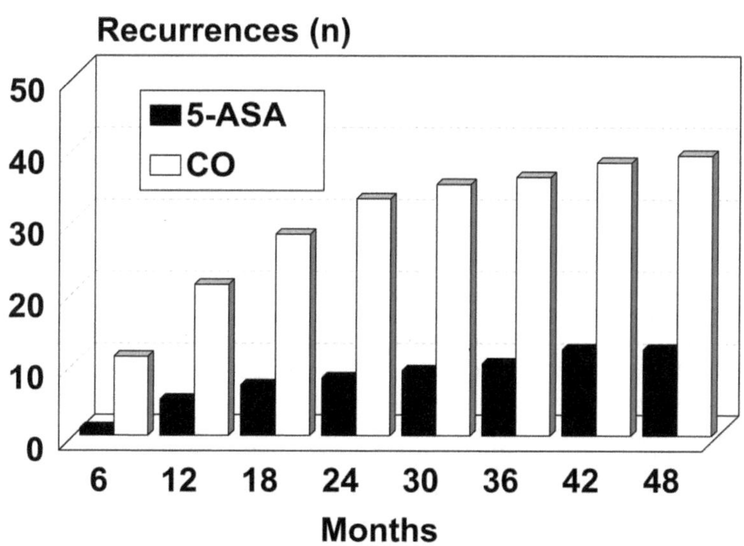

Figure 1 Symptomatic recurrence of diverticular disease[21]. Kaplan–Meier actuarial estimate. After an initial treatment with sulbactam/ampicillin and rifaximin patients were randomized to receive a supplementary treatment with 5-aminosalicylic acid (400 mg b.i.d.) or no other treatment from week 2 to 9. Eighty-one patients received 5-aminosalicylic acid, 85 patients no supplementary treatment. The patients were followed up for 4 years.

Tursi et al.[22] compared the efficacy of a combined treatment with rifaximin and mesalazine versus rifaximin alone in patients with recurrent attacks of diverticulitis. A total of 218 consecutive patients with diverticulitis were included in this study; 109 patients were treated with rifaximin (400 mg b.i.d. for 7 days followed by 400 mg b.i.d. for 7 days/month), while the other group of

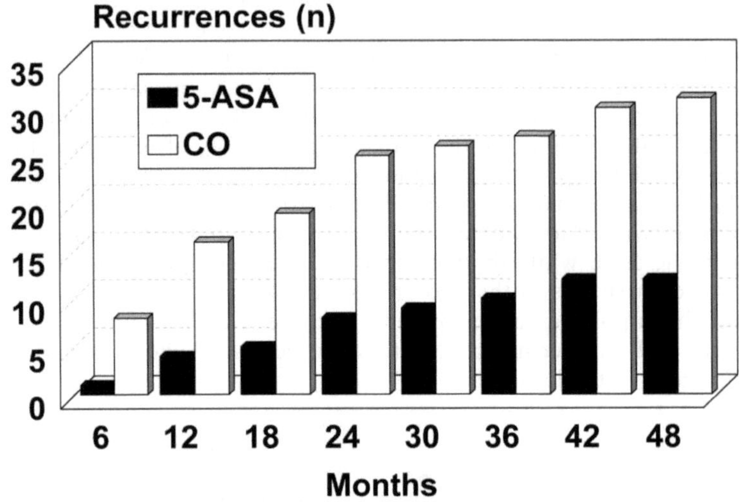

Figure 2 Recurrent minor diverticular haemorrhage[21]. Kaplan–Meier actuarial estimate. After an initial treatment with sulbactam/ampicillin and rifaximin patients were randomized to receive a supplementary treatment with 5-aminosalicylic acid (400 mg b.i.d.) or no other treatment from week 2 to 9. Eighty-one patients received 5-aminosalicylic acid, 85 patients no supplementary treatment. The patients were followed up for 4 years

109 patients was treated with rifaximin 400 mg b.i.d. plus 5-aminosalicylic acid 800 mg t.i.d. for 7 days, followed by rifaximin 400 mg b.i.d. plus 5-aminosalicylic acid 800 mg b.i.d. for 7 days/month. Follow-up was for 1 year. At the end of the follow-up 193 patients were fully compliant with the therapy. More patients were symptom-free in the combination treatment group (rifaximin plus 5-aminosalicylic acid) versus the rifaximin group after 3 months (44.4% vs 17.4%), after 6 months (63.0% vs 29.8%), after 9 months (73.8% vs 39.3%), and after 12 months (85.6% vs 49.4%) (Figure 3). In the combined treatment group more patients had regular bowel habits than in the rifaximin group (after 3 months 38.5% vs 17.4%, after 6 months 52.8% vs 31.7%, after 9 months 66.4% vs 47.4%, and after 12 months 78.9% vs 59.6%) (Figure 4). While three patients in the combined treatment group (2.75%) showed a recurrence of acute diverticulitis during the follow-up, this was the case for 16 patients in the rifaximin group (18.0%). The authors concluded from their study that rifaximin plus 5-aminosalicylic acid is more effective than rifaximin alone in the resolution of symptoms and the prevention of the recurrence of diverticulitis.

In a prospective study Brandimarte et al.[23] tested the effectiveness of a treatment with rifaximin/5-aminosalicylic acid followed by 5-aminosalicylic acid alone in 90 consecutive patients with uncomplicated diverticulitis. All patients were treated initially with rifaximin 800 mg/day plus 5-aminosalicylic acid 2.4 g/day for 10 days, followed by 5-aminosalicylic acid 1.6 g/day for 8

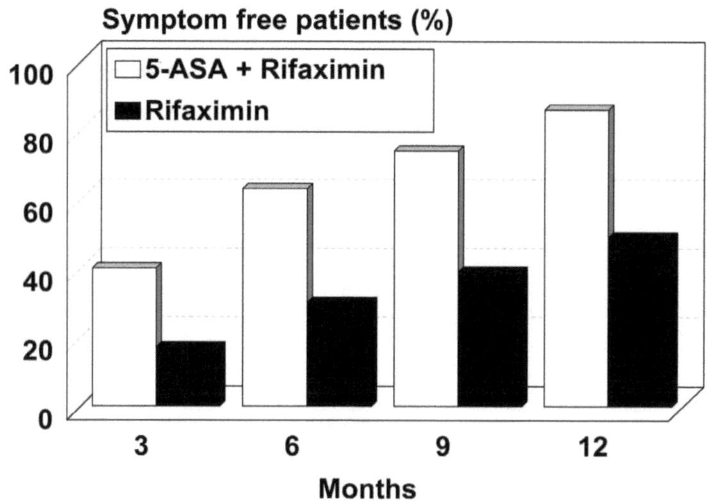

Figure 3 Symptom-free patients with previous recurrent attacks of diverticulitis[22]. A total of 218 patients with reccurent attacks of diverticulitis were treated initially with rifaximin (400 mg b.i.d. for 7 days followed by 400 mg b.i.d. for 7 days/month). 109 patients were treated with rifaximin 400 mg b.i.d. + 5-aminosalicylic acid 800 mg t.i.d. for 7 days followed by rifaximin 400 mg b.i.d. + 5-aminosalicylic acid 800 mg b.i.d. for 7 days/month. Follow-up was for 1 year

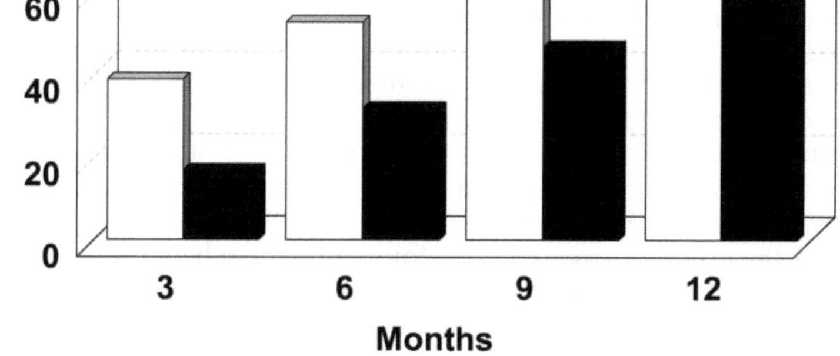

Figure 4 Patients with regular bowel habits and previous recurrent attacks of diverticulitis[22]. A total of 218 patients with recurrent attacks of diverticulitis were treated initially with rifaximin (400 mg b.i.d. for 7 days followed by 400 mg b.i.d. for 7 days/month), 109 patients were treated with rifaximin 400 mg b.i.d. + 5-aminosalicylic acid 800 mg t.i.d. for 7 days followed by rifaximin 400 mg b.i.d. + 5-aminosalicylic acid 800 mg b.i.d. for 7 days/month. Follow-up was for 1 year

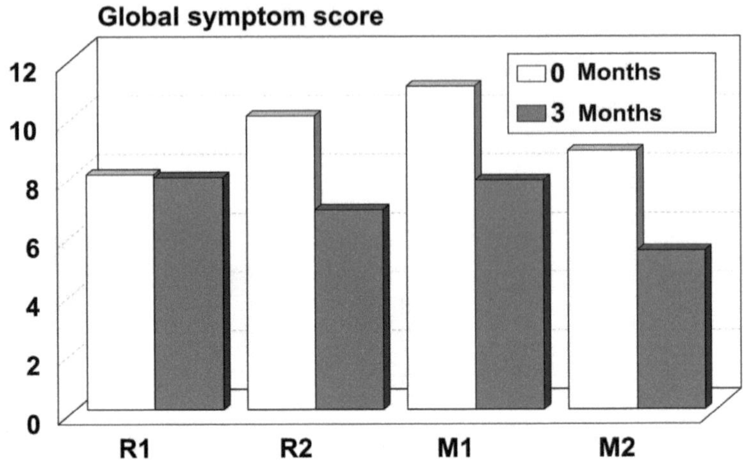

Figure 5 Global symptom score in patients with symptomatic diverticular disease[25]. One hundred and seventy patients with symptomatic and uncomplicated diverticular disease were enrolled in the trial and treated with four different schedules according to a randomization list: group R1 (39 patients) received rifaximin 200 mg b.i.d., group R2 (43 patients) received rifaximin 400 mg b.i.d., group M1 (40 patients) received mesalazine 400 mg b.i.d., group M2 (48 patients) received mesalazine 800 mg b.i.d. Each treatment was given for 10 days every month. The patients were evaluated at 0 and 3 months. Symptoms were assessed with 11 clinical variables (upper abdominal pain/discomfort, lower abdominal pain/discomfort, bloating, tenesmus, diarrhoea, abdominal tenderness, fever, general illness, nausea, emesis, dysuria)

weeks. The patients were re-evaluated at the end of the 8-week treatment with 5-aminosalicylic acid. Eighty-six patients were completely asymptomatic after 8 weeks of treatment with 5-aminosalicylic acid alone. Two patients showed recurrence of symptoms and two patients developed diarrhoea. The authors concluded that rifaximin/5-aminosalicylic acid followed by 5-aminosalicylic acid alone is extremely effective in obtaining the resolution of symptoms in patients with uncomplicated diverticulitis.

The aim of another study was to evaluate the efficacy of 5-aminosalicylic acid in the relief of symptoms in patients with symptomatic and uncomplicated diverticular disease[24]. Two hundred and forty-eight consecutive patients were enrolled in the trial and treated with four different schedules according to a randomization list: group R1 (57 patients) received rifaximin 200 mg b.i.d., group R2 (69 patients) received rifaximin 400 mg b.i.d., group M1 (60 patients) received mesalazine 400 mg b.i.d., group M2 (62 patients) received mesalazine 800 mg b.i.d. Each treatment was given for 10 days every month. The patients were evaluated every 3 months for up to a year. Symptoms were assessed with 11 clinical variables (upper abdominal pain/discomfort, lower abdominal pain/discomfort, bloating, tenesmus, diarrhoea, abdominal tenderness, fever, general illness, nausea, emesis, dysuria). After 3, 6 and 12 months of follow-up patients treated with mesalazine (groups M1 and M2 together) showed a lower global symptom score as compared to patients treated with rifaximin (groups R1 and R2 together). The authors concluded from their study that the cyclic administration of mesalazine is effective in obtaining symptom relief in uncomplicated diverticular disease.

Earlier results of the above-mentioned study have recently been published as a full paper[25]. The numbers of patients in the various treatment groups were smaller (R1: $n = 39$, R2: $n = 43$, M1: $n = 40$, M: $n = 48$) and the follow-up time was only 3 months. After 3 months all groups but group R1 had a significantly reduced lower global symptom score (Figure 5).

CONCLUSION

Due to the broad spectrum of anti-inflammatory activity of aminosalicylates there is a rationale for their use in symptomatic diverticular disease. The available data of four open studies suggest that mesalazine may have favourable effects in symptomatic diverticular disease. These findings should therefore be confirmed in well-designed placebo-controlled randomized clinical trials.

References

1. Ligumsky M, Karmeli F, Sharon P, Zor U, Cohen F, Rachmilewitz D. Enhanced thromboxane A2 and prostacyclin production by cultured rectal mucosa in ulcerative colitis and its inhibition by steroids and sulfasalazine. Gastroenterology. 1981;81:444–9.
2. Sharon P, Ligumsky M, Rachmilewitz D, Zor U. Role of prostaglandins in ulcerative colitis – enhanced production during active disease and inhibition by sulfasalazine. Gastroenterology. 1978;75:638–40.
3. Keating JJ, Maxwell WJ, Hogan FP, Keeling PWN. Effects of prednisolone, sulphasalazine, 5-aminosalicylic acid and indomethacin on prostaglandin E2 and leucotrine B4 production. Jubilee Meeting of the British Society of Gastroenterology, London, 15–18 September 1987: Abstract Th79.
4. Greenfield SM, Boswell DJ, Punchard NA, Thompson RPH. The effects of 5-aminosalicylic acid and acetyl-5-aminosalicylic acid on lipid peroxidation in erythrocytes and prostaglandin production by mononuclear cells. Aliment Pharmacol Ther. 1992;6:671–83.
5. Lauritsen K, Laursen LS, Bukhave K, Rask-Madsen J. Effect of topical 5-aminosalicylic acid and prednisolone on prostaglandin E2 and leukotriene B4 levels determined by equilibrium *in vivo* dialysis of rectum in relapsing ulcerative colitis. Gastroenterology. 1986;91:837–44.
6. Nielsen OH, Bukhave K, Elmgreen J, Ahnfeldt-Rønne I. Inhibition of 5-lipoxygenase pathway of arachidonic acid metabolism in human neutrophils by sulfasalazine and 5-aminosalicylic acid. Dig Dis Sci. 1987;32:577–82.
7. Peskar BM, Dreyling KW, May B, Schaarschmidt K, Goebell H. Possible mode of action of 5-aminosalicylic acid. Dig Dis Sci. 1987;32(Suppl):S51–6.
8. Allgayer H, Höfer P, Schmidt M, Böhne P, Kruis W, Gugler R. Superoxide hydroxyl and fatty acid radical scavenging by aminosalicylates – direct evaluation with electron spin resonance spectroscopy. Biochem Pharmacol. 1992;43:259–62.
9. Gionchetti P, Guarnieri C, Campieri M et al. Scavenger effect of sulfasalazine, 5-aminosalicylic acid, and olsalazine on superoxide radical generation. Dig Dis Sci. 1991;36: 174–8.
10. Miyachi Y, Yoshioka A, Imamura S, Niwa Y. Effect of sulphasalazine and its metabolites on the generation of reactive oxygen species. Gut. 1987;28:190–5.

11. Ahnfeldt-Rønne I, Nielsen OH, Christensen A, Langholz E, Binder V, Riis P. Clinical evidence supporting the radical scavenger mechanism of 5-aminosalicylic acid. Gastroenterology. 1990;98:38–41.
12. Mahida YR, Lamming CED, Gallagher A, Hawthorne AB, Hawkey CJ. 5-Aminosalicylic acid is a potent inhibitor of interleukin 1 beta production in organ culture of colonic biopsy specimens from patients with inflammatory bowel disease. Gut. 1991;32:50–4.
13. Rachmilewitz D, Karmeli F, Schwartz LW, Simon PL. Effect of aminophenols (5-ASA and 4-ASA) on colonic interleukin-1 generation. Gut. 1992;33:929–32.
14. Greenfield SM, Hamblin AS, Shakoor ZS, Teare JP, Punchard NA, Thompson RPH. Inhibition of leucocyte adhesion molecule upregulation by tumor necrosis factor α: a novel mechanism of action of sulphasalazine. Gut. 1993;34:252–6.
15. Rachmilewitz D, Eliakim R, Simon P, Ligumsky M, Karmeli F. Role of cytokines and platelet activating factor in the pathogenesis of inflammatory bowel disease. In: Goebell H, Malchow H, Ewe K, Koelbel C, editors. Inflammatory Bowel Disease – Progress in Basic Research and Clinical Implications. Dordrecht: Kluwer, 1991:153–9.
16. Molin L, Stendahl O. The effect of sulfasalazine and its active components on human polymorphonuclear leukocyte function in relation to ulcerative colitis. Acta Med Scand. 1979;206:451–7.
17. Rhodes JM, Bartholomew TC, Jewell DP. Inhibition of leucocyte motility by drugs used in ulcerative colitis. Gut. 1981;22:642–7.
18. Wandall JH. Effects of sulphasalazine and its metabolites on neutrophil chemotaxis, superoxide production, degranulation and translocation of cytochrome b-245. Aliment Pharmacol Ther. 1991;5:609–19.
19. Fox CC, Moore WC, Lichtenstein LM. Modulation of mediator release from human intestinal mast cells by sulfasalazine and 5-aminosalicylic acid. Dig Dis Sci. 1991;36:179–84.
20. Shah PM, Boulos PB, Pearce F. The effect of sulphasalazine and its metabolites on histamine release from human colonic and gastric mast cells. Agents Actions. 1993;38 (Special Conference Issue): C194–6.
21. Trespi E, Colla C, Panizza P et al. Therapeutic and prophylactic role of mesalazine (5-ASA) in symptomatic diverticular disease of the colon. Minverva Gastroenterol Dietol. 1999;45: 245–52.
22. Tursi A, Brandimarte G, Daffina R. Long-term treatment with mesalazine and rifaximin versus rifaximin alone for patients with recurrent attacks of acute diverticulitis of colon. Digest Liver Dis. 2002;34:510–15
23. Brandimarte G, Tursi A, Elisei W, Annunziata V, Villa S. Rifaximin/mesalazine followed by mesalazine alone is highly effective in obtaining remission of uncomplicated diverticulitis of colon. Dig Liver Dis. 2004;36:S202.
24. Aragona G, Leandro G, Fanigliulo L et al. Efficacy of mesalazine in the treatment of symptomatic diverticular disease. Gastroenterology. 2004;126(Supp. 2):A253.
25. Di Mario F, Aragona G, Leandro G et al. Efficacy of mesalazine in the treatment of symptomatic diverticular disease. Dig Dis Sci 2005;50:581–6.

Section IX
Treatment – miscellaneous

Chair: J. MÖSSNER and D. ÖRTLI

22
Diverticular disease: persistent symptoms after surgery

M. K. PETER, D. CANDINAS and B. EGGER

EPIDEMIOLOGY AND PATHOPHYSIOLOGY

In Western countries the prevalence of diverticular disease has increased over the past century[1]. This probably reflects both an increase in detection and an ageing population. Prevalence of diverticular disease increases with age, from less than 10% in people younger than age 40 years to 50–66% in patients older than age 80 years[2–4]. Studies from the 1970s and 1980s related its occurrence to the use of low-fibre diets and to the prolonged colonic transit time and increased intraluminal pressure associated with low-volume stools. The incidence of complicated diverticulitis has risen up to 50% in the past two decades, an increase attributed to an ageing population and reduced fibre consumption[5]. Furthermore, patients with symptomatic diverticulosis have also been shown to have higher motility indices than either asymptomatic patients or healthy controls[6], which may be another important pathogenetic factor. Pseudodiverticula emerge through the thickened circular layer of the muscularis propria of the left colon at points of penetration of the vasa recta that supply the submucosa and mucosa. In numbers, diverticula range from solitary findings to many hundreds. Most are single, located in the sigmoid colon, and asymptomatic, but can present with infection and its complications such as haemorrhage, abscess formation, obstruction, fistula and free perforation[7].

NATURAL HISTORY AND SYMPTOMS

Most patients with diverticulosis will remain asymptomatic throughout their lifetime. Of the ones who develop symptoms (10–25%)[4], diverticulitis and its complications such as perforation, abscesses, fistulas, or obstruction, is the most common clinical manifestation followed by diverticular haemorrhage. However, patients may also present with non-specific abdominal complaints such as lower left-sided abdominal pain, abdominal distension or episodes of diarrhoea. Such symptoms may last for years while patients do not develop clinical signs of inflammation which could indicate diverticulitis. Symptoms may be exacerbated by eating, and diminished with defaecation or flatus, which suggests colonic wall tension due to raised intraluminal pressure. Patients might also complain about other symptoms such as extensive bloating or severe constipation.

DIAGNOSIS

Barium enema, which has been the standard diagnostic investigation in diverticulosis patients for years, is currently replaced by colonoscopy. Extensive clinical experience has shown that colonoscopy is safe in this population, although after a history of diverticulitis the colon can be difficult to examine because of spasm, luminal narrowing, and fixation[8]. Today, in patients with suspected diverticulitis, computed tomography scanning with intravenous, oral, and rectal contrast is regarded as the diagnostic procedure of choice[9,10].

TREATMENT

Patients with diagnosed uncomplicated diverticulitis should be treated – as inpatients or outpatients, depending on the severity of the disease – with a clear liquid diet and broad-spectrum antibiotics with activity against anaerobes and Gram-negative bacteria for 7–10 days. Most patients treated for acute diverticulitis will respond to conservative treatment, but 15–30% will need surgery during that time[11–13]. Abscesses may be drained percutaneously by interventional radiology but free perforation with generalized peritonitis still requires urgent surgical intervention[12,13]. For most patients who respond well to conservative treatment, an important clinical question is the role of prophylactic resection in order to prevent further recurrences. Since symptoms after an attack of acute diverticulitis recur in between 7% and 45%, and are less likely to respond to conservative treatment with considerable mortality rate[11,12], most experts agree that elective resection is indicated after two attacks of uncomplicated diverticulitis[14–16]. In the surgical management laparoscopic intervention of sigmoid diverticular disease has emerged as an important adjunct. The increasingly favourable experiences with this surgical technique in the hands of skilled laparoscopic surgeons may soon be sufficient to make laparoscopic colectomy the standard procedure of choice[17–21].

RECURRENT DIVERTICULITIS

The rate of recurrent diverticulitis following resection of the sigmoid colon ranges between 1% and 10%[22–26]. The correlation between recurrence rates and extent of bowel resection and/or level of anastomosis above the anus may be still considered an unclear issue in surgery for uncomplicated diverticulitis of the sigmoid. Wolff et al.[27] have reported that the rates of recurrent diverticulitis after conventional surgery do not depend on the number of proximal diverticula. Benn et al.[23] demonstrated that recurrence rate is decreased significantly when the distal line of resection is placed on the rectum instead of the distal sigmoid colon. In cases of a laparoscopic approach, there are few data to conclude definitively on long-term recurrence rates due to short follow-up time[28]. However, Thaler et al.[29] were recently able to show in a 5-year follow-up study that surgical access to sigmoid resection (laparoscopic or open) for uncomplicated sigmoid diverticulitis is unlikely to have an impact on recurrence rates provided that the oral bowel end is anastomosed to the proximal rectum rather than to the distal sigmoid.

PERSISTING SYMPTOMS

Some patients will still have symptoms other than recurrent diverticulitis following resection of the sigmoid colon. Persisting symptoms following surgery form one reason, which casts doubts on recommendations to proceed to elective surgery after experiencing two attacks of acute diverticulitis. This topic is extensively addressed in a recently published review by Janes et al.[30]. In brief, there are conflicting results which indicate a weak association between histological and clinical findings. Breen et al.[31] reported 100 consecutive elective resections for presumed diverticular disease, showing that 24% of resected specimens had no histological evidence of acute or chronic inflammation. During a mean follow-up of 37 months, 60% of patients with no histological inflammation experienced a range of continuing symptoms, whereas only 15% of those with inflammation were symptomatic during follow-up. Patients symptomatic for more than 1 year before surgery were also significantly less likely to be asymptomatic during follow-up. Moreaux and Vons[32] reported similar findings in a 21-year retrospective review of 177 interventions for complicated diverticular disease. Patients without histological evidence of inflammation were seven times more likely to experience persistent postoperative symptoms and twice as likely to have recurrent diverticulitis as those with histological inflammation. Additionally, irritable bowel syndrome associated with diverticular disease may explain a higher rate of unsatisfactory results[32,33]. Depending on diagnostic criteria, the prevalence of irritable bowel syndrome is up to 14% in patients with diverticular disease[34]; therefore some individuals may have symptoms attributable to both conditions. Munson et al.[35] reported that, even after sigmoid resection for histologically proven diverticulitis, 27% of patients experienced ongoing abdominal symptoms. All of these patients undergoing sigmoid resection stated that localization of symptoms was the same as before the operation. Character of pain was unchanged in two-thirds and one-third complained of pain characteristics being completely changed compared with the preoperative pain. The authors concluded that the reasons for these symptoms are poorly understood, and may simply represent coexisting irritable bowel syndrome.

PERSONAL EXPERIENCE

We have also evaluated the data of our own patients' series from our prospective database on patients who have been consecutively operated for diverticular disease from 1999 to 2004. A total of 162 patients (80 females, 82 males) with a mean age of 63 (28–96) years have been operated on for diverticular disease within this 5-year period. All patients have been operated by a standardized intervention with resection of the rectosigmoid colon (>20 cm) and with an inferior resection line in the proximal rectum. A total of 124 (77%) patients could be contacted for follow-up (median age 61 (28–89) years) with a mean follow up time of 33 (4–72) months; 23 (14%) died in the meantime and 15 (9%) were lost to follow-up. Of these 124 patients 55% underwent elective and 45% emergency operation. Recurrent diverticulitis was observed in two (1.6%) patients and was successfully treated in a conservative manner in both. Of our patients 30 (24%) complained of persistent symptoms at the time of follow-up. Symptoms were constipation in 11 (36.7%), abdominal distension in seven (23.3%), crampy abdominal pain in seven (23.3%) and diarrhoea in seven (23.3%) patients. All patients with either recurrent diverticulitis or persisting symptoms were treated conservatively. At the time of the last follow-up quality of life concerning the surgical intervention was very good in 51%, good in 42%, moderate in 6% and bad in 1% of patients. In a specific scale system, no significant differences in persistent symptoms were found when comparing elective and emergency, as well as comparing open and laparoscopically operated patients.

CONCLUSIONS

The rate of recurrent diverticulitis is low provided that the oral bowel end is anastomosed to the proximal rectum rather than to the distal sigmoid. However, following successful surgical treatment of diverticular disease, there remains a significant group with mild but persistent symptoms different from recurrent diverticulitis. In the literature there is scant information about the symptoms these patients experience after surgery. Thirty-five years ago Parks and Connell[36] first reported on this problem. They found that 24% of patients treated with a three-stage procedure continued to have mild symptoms. However, sources of symptoms were not well defined in this study. Some 9 years ago Munson et al.[35] reported 27% of their surgically treated patients to have persistent symptoms, especially ongoing abdominal pain. In our own patients series we have found 24% of resected patients with mild persistent symptoms, such as abdominal distension, crampy abdominal pain, constipation or diarrhoea. The reason for these ongoing symptoms is poorly understood and may well be related to other coexistent diseases such as irritable bowel syndrome. Patients undergoing resection need to be aware of this problem. Preoperative counselling and informed consent should also reflect the possibility of persisting symptoms after surgery. In all cases patients should be informed that surgery may not completely relieve their symptoms.

References

1. Hughes LE. Postmortem survey of diverticular disease of the colon. I. Diverticulosis and diverticulitis. Gut. 1969;10:336–44.
2. Painter NS, Burkitt DP. Diverticular disease of the colon: a deficiency disease of Western civilization. Br Med J. 1971;2:450–4.
3. Painter NS, Burkitt DP. Diverticular disease of the colon, a 20th century problem. Clin Gastroenterol. 1975;4:3–21.
4. Parks TG. Natural history of diverticular disease of the colon. Clin Gastroenterol. 1975;4: 53–69.
5. Makela J, Kiviniemi H, Laitinen S. Prevalence of perforated sigmoid diverticulitis is increasing. Dis Colon Rectum. 2002;45:955–61.
6. Cortesini C, Pantalone D. Usefulness of colonic motility study in identifying patients at risk for complicated diverticular disease. Dis Colon Rectum. 1991;34:339–42.
7. Levi DM, Levi JU, Rogers AI, Bergau DK, Wenger J. Giant colonic diverticulum: an unusual manifestation of a common disease. Am J Gastroenterol. 1993;88:139–42.
8. Anderson JC, Messina CR, Cohn W et al. Factors predictive of difficult colonoscopy. Gastrointest Endosc. 2001;54:558–62.
9. Ambrosetti P, Jenny A, Becker C, Terrier TF, Morel P. Acute left colonic diverticulitis – compared performance of computed tomography and water-soluble contrast enema: prospective evaluation of 420 patients. Dis Colon Rectum. 2000;43:1363–7.
10. Shrier D, Skucas J, Weiss S. Diverticulitis: an evaluation by computed tomography and contrast enema. Am J Gastroenterol. 1991;86:1466–71.
11. Parks TG. Natural history of diverticular disease of the colon. A review of 521 cases. Br Med J. 1969;4:639–42.
12. Roberts P, Abel M, Rosen L et al. Practice parameters for sigmoid diverticulitis. The Standards Task Force American Society of Colon and Rectal Surgeons. Dis Colon Rectum. 1995;38:125–32.
13. Roberts PL, Veidenheimer MC. Current management of diverticulitis. Adv Surg. 1994;27: 189–208.
14. Kohler L, Sauerland S, Neugebauer E. Diagnosis and treatment of diverticular disease: results of a consensus development conference. Scientific Committee of the European Association for Endoscopic Surgery. Surg Endosc. 1999;13:430–6.
15. Stollman NH, Raskin JB. Diagnosis and management of diverticular disease of the colon in adults. Ad Hoc Practice Parameters Committee of the American College of Gastroenterology. Am J Gastroenterol. 1999;94:3110–21.
16. Wong WD, Wexner SD, Lowry A et al. Practice parameters for the treatment of sigmoid diverticulitis – supporting documentation. Standards Task Force. American Society of Colon and Rectal Surgeons. Dis Colon Rectum. 2000;43:290–7.
17. Degiuli M, Mineccia M, Bertone A et al. Outcome of laparoscopic colorectal resection. Surg Endosc. 2004;18:427–32.
18. Lawrence DM, Pasquale MD, Wasser TE. Laparoscopic versus open sigmoid colectomy for diverticulitis. Am Surg. 2003;69:499–503.
19. Natarajan S, Ewings EL, Vega RJ. Laparoscopic sigmoid colectomy after acute diverticulitis: when to operate? Surgery. 2004;136:725–30.
20. Scheidbach H, Schneider C, Rose J et al. Laparoscopic approach to treatment of sigmoid diverticulitis: changes in the spectrum of indications and results of a prospective, multicenter study on 1545 patients. Dis Colon Rectum. 2004;47:1883–8.
21. Schwandner O, Farke S, Fischer F, Eckmann C, Schiedeck TH, Bruch HP. Laparoscopic colectomy for recurrent and complicated diverticulitis: a prospective study of 396 patients. Langenbecks Arch Surg. 2004;389:97–103.
22. Bacon HE, Berkley JL. The surgical management of diverticulitis of the colon with particular reference to rehabilitation. Arch Surg. 1960;80:646–9.
23. Benn PL, Wolff BG, Ilstrup DM. Level of anastomosis and recurrent colonic diverticulitis. Am J Surg. 1986;151:269–71.
24. Farmakis N, Tudor RG, Keighley MR. The 5-year natural history of complicated diverticular disease. Br J Surg. 1994;81:733–5.
25. Leigh JE, Judd ES, Waugh JM. Diverticulitis of the colon. Recurrence after apparently adequate segmental resection. Am J Surg. 1962;103:51–4.

26. Marsh J, Liem RK, Byrd BF Jr, Daniel RA. One hundred consecutive operations for diverticulitis of the colon. South Med J. 1975;68:133–7.
27. Wolff BG, Ready RL, MacCarty RL, Dozois RR, Beart RW Jr. Influence of sigmoid resection on progression of diverticular disease of the colon. Dis Colon Rectum. 1984;27: 645–7.
28. Bergamaschi R, Arnaud JP. Anastomosis level and specimen length in surgery for uncomplicated diverticulitis of the sigmoid. Surg Endosc. 1998;12:1149–51.
29. Thaler K, Weiss EG, Nogueras JJ, Arnaud JP, Wexner SD, Bergamaschi R. Recurrence rates at minimum five-year follow-up: laparoscopic versus open sigmoid resection for uncomplicated diverticulitis. Acta Chir Iugosl. 2004;51:45–7.
30. Janes S, Meagher A, Frizelle FA. Elective surgery after acute diverticulitis. Br J Surg. 2005; 92:133–42.
31. Breen RE, Corman ML, Robertson WG, Prager ED. Are we really operating on diverticulitis? Dis Colon Rectum. 1986;29:174–6.
32. Moreaux J, Vons C. Elective resection for diverticular disease of the sigmoid colon. Br J Surg 1990;77:1036–8.
33. Thorn M, Graf W, Stefansson T, Pahlman L. Clinical and functional results after elective colonic resection in 75 consecutive patients with diverticular disease. Am J Surg. 2002;183: 7–11.
34. Simpson J, Neal KR, Scholefield JH, Spiller RC. Patterns of pain in diverticular disease and the influence of acute diverticulitis. Eur J Gastroenterol Hepatol. 2003;15:1005–10.
35. Munson KD, Hensien MA, Jacob LN, Robinson AM, Liston WA. Diverticulitis. A comprehensive follow-up. Dis Colon Rectum 1996;39:318–22.
36. Parks TG, Connell AM. The outcome in 455 patients admitted for treatment of diverticular disease of the colon. Br J Surg. 1970;57:775–8.

23
Primary and secondary prevention of diverticular disease

W. H. ALDOORI

INTRODUCTION

Diverticular disease (DD) is one of the most common disorders of the colon among the elderly in the Western world. The prevalence of DD is difficult to measure, because between 70% and 80% of patients are asymptomatic; however, it is well recognized that the prevalence of DD increases with ageing. It is estimated that DD affects about 10% of those younger than 40 years and this prevalence increases to affect between 50% and 66% of those older than 80 years[1–5]. Despite an earlier report that DD is more prevalent among women[6], results of recent studies indicate that there are no differences by gender[7–9]. Although the condition is mainly asymptomatic in the majority of cases, it is estimated that 10–25% of affected individuals develop symptoms[10]. Symptomatic diverticular disease results in 200 000 hospitalizations in the USA annually[11], and this number is expected to increase with the growing number of seniors in the population. According to a recent report by the American Gastroenterological Association, DD is the fifth most important gastrointestinal disease in terms of direct and indirect costs, with a mortality rate of 2.5 per 100 000 per year[12]. Earlier this century DD was widely believed to be extremely rare, and was regarded as a pathological curiosity. This prompted Burkitt and Painter to call it 'a 20th century problem' or 'a disease of Western civilization'[2,4], in contrast to its rarity in many developing countries[13]. The main explanation for the increase in the prevalence of DD was largely attributed to dietary changes, mainly due to the decline of dietary fibre intake, particularly cereal fibre[4]. Recent evidence indicates that there is a rapid increase in the prevalence of DD in many developing countries, which could be attributed to urbanization and /or lifestyle changes[14–16]. This suggests that lifestyle factors such as diet might partially explain this increase.

Three decades have passed since the fibre hypothesis was widely publicized. The dietary fibre hypothesis was earlier supported by human[17–22] and animal studies[23–25]. Previous case–control studies have consistently found that patients diagnosed with diverticula report lower fibre intake than controls. However, the findings of case–control studies were related to the diet mainly after the onset of symptoms, which may have been altered as a result of the disease[21]. In addition, failure to control for potential risk factors – such as physical activity, alcohol, smoking, coffee drinking, and other dietary component and non-dietary factors – limits the interpretation of most case–control studies[26]. Therefore we studied, prospectively, the association between crude fibre, total dietary fibre and sources of fibre (vegetable, cereal, fruit, soluble, insoluble, cellulose, hemicellulose, and lignin) other dietary components (e.g. red meat, fats, different dietary sources of fat, alcohol and caffeine consumption), non-dietary factors (e.g. physical activity, body composition, smoking, and analgesic use) and the diagnosis of DD among US men participating in the Health Professionals Follow-up Study (HPFS)[27–31]. To our knowledge the HPFS is the first, and at present the only, prospective study investigating the association between the above-mentioned factors and the risk of DD. The prospective design of this study makes the findings more compelling than case–control studies because dietary and non-dietary information was collected before the diagnosis of DD.

This chapter reviews in particular our experience in investigating the association between dietary and non-dietary factors and the risk of DD with special emphasis on the prevention of this condition.

HEALTH PROFESSIONALS FOLLOW-UP STUDY (HPFS)

Details about the HPFS, exposure assessment, identification of DD cases and statistical methods were published earlier[27–31]. Briefly, the HPFS is a prospective study of heart disease and cancer among 51 529 US male health professionals, residing in 50 US states and aged 40–75 years in 1986. The study population consists of 29 683 dentists, 3745 optometrists, 2218 osteopathic physicians, 4185 pharmacists, 1600 podiatrists, and 10 098 veterinarians. This ongoing study began in 1986 when cohort members completed a detailed food-frequency questionnaire and provided other relevant information. Every 2 years follow-up questionnaires have been sent to update information on potential risk factors and to identify newly diagnosed cases of various diseases, as well as reassessing the diet every 4 years. To reduce the possibility of detection bias we used symptomatic DD as our primary endpoint. We considered the cases ascertained during the 4 years of follow-up – between 1 February, 1988 and 31 January 31, 1992.

DIETARY FACTORS AND THE RISK OF DD

Dietary fibre and fibre types

The dietary fibre hypothesis, dietary fibre sources or fibre types were not previously investigated prospectively. In our prospective study the intakes of crude and total dietary fibre were both inversely associated with the risk of DD in the age- and energy-adjusted analysis. These findings did not change appreciably after adjustments for other potentially confounding variables (Table 1).

Table 1 Relative risk of DD by quintiles of total dietary fibre, crude fibre, and by dietary fibre from fruits, vegetables and cereals (from ref. 27)

Variable	*Quintile* 1	2	3	4	5	*p-Value for trend*
Vegetable fibre (median g/day)	3.4	5.1	6.6	8.6	12.4	
Cases	84	82	87	78		
RR† (95% CI)	1.0	0.93 (0.68–1.28)	0.98 (0.71–1.35)	0.90 (0.64–1.26)	0.55 (0.37-0.84)	0.003
Multivariate RR‡ (95% CI)	1.0	0.96 (0.70–1.31)	1.0 (0.73–1.36)	0.87 (0.63–1.20)	0.59 (0.41–0.86)	0.003
Cereal fibre (median g/day)	1.7	3.7	5.7	8.2	13.5	
Cases	77	91	78	61	78	
RR† (95% CI)	1.0	1.21 (0.89–1.66)	1.10 (0.79–1.54)	0.85 (0.58–1.24)	1.09 (0.77–1.54)	0.23
Multivariate RR‡ (95% CI)	1.0	1.23 (0.90–1.67)	1.08 (0.78–1.49)	0.87 (0.61–1.22)	1.06 (0.76–1.47)	0.72
Total dietary fibre (median g/day)	13.0	18.0	21.0	24.0	32.0	
Cases	99	75	73	83	55	
RR† (95% CI)	1.0	0.76 (0.57–1.03)	0.73 (0.54–0.99)	0.78 (0.58–1.05)	0.51 (0.37–0.71)	0.0002
Multivariate RR‡ (95% CI)	1.0	0.79 (0.58–1.07)	0.77 (0.57–1.05)	0.87 (0.64–1.17)	0.58 (0.41–0.83)	0.01
Total crude fibre (median g/day)	3.3	4.5	5.4	6.4	8.3	
Cases	101	72	86	72	54	
RR† (95% CI)	1.0	0.78 (0.58–1.06)	0.72 (0.54–0.96)	0.71 (0.52–0.96)	0.48 (0.35–0.67)	<0.00001
Multivariate RR‡ (95% CI)	1.0	0.81 (0.59–1.10)	0.76 (0.57–1.02)	0.78 (0.57–1.06)	0.54 (0.38–0.76)	0.01
Fruit fibre (median g/day)	1.1	2.3	3.8	5.5	8.8	
Cases	85	98	84	57	61	
RR† (95% CI)	1.0	1.03 (0.77–1.38)	0.85 (0.63–1.15)	0.54 (0.39–.076)	0.62 (0.45–0.86)	<0.00001
Multivariate RR‡ (95% CI)	1.0	1.10 (0.82–1.47)	0.90 (0.66–1.23)	0.60 (0.43–0.85)	0.61 (0.43–0.87)	<0.00001

*Test for trend was calculated by using the median intake of nutrients in each quintile as a continuous variable in a multiple logistic regression.

†Adjusted for age and total energy.

‡Adjusted for age, physical activity, and energy-adjusted total fat. CI denotes confidence interval.

We computed the contribution of age- and energy-adjusted dietary fibre from fruits, vegetables, and cereals. Intake of fruit and vegetable fibre was inversely associated with risk of DD (Table 1). Cereal fibre was not associated with a decreased risk of DD (Table 1). However, after adjusting for age and total energy, intake of bran added to food was inversely associated with the risk of DD (relative risk (RR) for five or more tablespoons/week = 0.59, 95% CI 0.36–0.98), but this association was not statistically significant (*p* for trend = 0.13).

When we analysed separately the sources of dietary fibre (fruits, vegetables, or cereals) in multivariate models including age, total energy intake, total fat, and physical activity, our findings for each source of dietary fibre did not change appreciably from those in the age- and energy-adjusted model (Table 1). When we included these three sources of dietary fibre (fruits, vegetables, and cereals) simultaneously in the multivariate model with age, total energy intake, total fat, and physical activity, our findings did not change appreciably (RR for fruit fibre = 0.66, 95% CI 0.46–0.95, RR for vegetable fibre = 0.68, 95% CI 0.46–0.99, RR for cereal fibre = 1.18, 95% CI 0.85–1.65 for the highest quintile).

In our data fibre from fruit and vegetable sources, and not from cereal sources, was associated with a reduced risk of DD. Fibre from unprocessed cereal grains (mainly bran) is used in the treatment of DD, because it increases water-holding capacity, decreases faecal transit time, and increases faecal output, hence reducing constipation which is commonly associated with DD. In our study several of the dietary sources of cereal fibre were highly processed and are expected to have a minimal mechanical effect on colonic transit or pressure. Coarse milled bran was repeatedly shown to be more beneficial for colonic functions than finely milled bran[32–34]. This observation appears to be related to coarse bran physicochemical properties on faecal bulk, faecal water and its influence on colonic transit and pressure. Despite being chemically identical, fine bran provided none of those benefits[32–34].

Little is known about which specific dietary fibre components are associated with reduced risk of DD. In our study age- and energy-adjusted intakes of soluble fibre, insoluble fibre, cellulose, hemicellulose, and lignin were inversely associated with risk of DD (Tables 2 and 3). This association was particularly stronger for cellulose, lignin and insoluble fibre (Tables 2 and 3). When we analysed separately these sources of dietary fibre in multivariate models including age, energy-adjusted total fat, and physical activity, our findings for each source of dietary fibre did not change appreciably from those in the age- and energy-adjusted model (Tables 2 and 3). When we included soluble and insoluble fibre simultaneously in the multivariate model, the association with insoluble fibre did not change appreciably, but that with soluble fibre was eliminated (RR for insoluble fibre = 0.53, 95% CI 0.33–0.85, RR for soluble fibre = 1.34, 95% CI 0. 83–2.18, for the highest quintile). Similarly when we included hemicellulose, cellulose, and lignin in the multivariate model, the association with cellulose did not change appreciably, but that with hemicellulose and lignin was attenuated (RR for hemicellulose = 1.26, 95% CI 0.81–1.96, RR for cellulose = 0.57, 95% CI 0.34–0.94, RR for lignin = 0.80, 95% CI 0.47–1.38 for the highest quintile).

Table 2 Relative risk of DD by quintiles of soluble and insoluble fibre components (adapted from ref. 30)

Variable	*Quintile*					*p-Value for trend*
	1	*2*	*3*	*4*	*5*	
Soluble fibre (g/day)	4.10	5.10	5.90	9.90	8.60	
RR* (95% CI)	1.0	1.03 (0.75–1.43)	1.00 (0.72–1.38)	0.83 (0.59–1.17)	0.82 (0.59–1.16)	0.05
Multivariate RR† (95% CI)	1.0	1.05 (0.76–1.45)	1.04 (0.75–1.44)	0.91 (0.65–1.29)	0.90 (0.62–1.29)	0.40
Insoluble fibre (g/day)	10.1	13.0	15.20	17.90	22.70	
RR* (95% CI)	1.0	0.89 (0.65–1.22)	0.78 (0.57–1.07)	0.80 (0.59–1.10)	0.55 (0.39–0.78)	0.001
Multivariate RR† (95% CI)	1.0	0.91 (0.66–1.24)	0.80 (0.58–1.10)	0.87 (0.63–1.20)	0.63 (0.44–0.91)	0.02

*Adjusted for age and total energy. CI denotes confidence interval.

†Adjusted for age, physical activity, and energy-adjusted total fat.

Table 3 Relative risk of DD by quintiles of hemicellulose, cellulose, and lignin intake (adapted from ref. 30)

Variable	*Quintile* 1	2	3	4	5	*p-Value for trend**
Hemicellulose (g/day)	4.40	6.00	7.30	8.90	11.70	
RR* (95% CI)	1.0	1.27 (0.94–1.71)	0.77 (0.55–1.07)	0.78 (0.56–1.09)	0.78 (0.56–1.08)	0.01
Multivariate RR† (95% CI)	1.0	1.29 (0.95–1.74)	0.79 (0.56–1.10)	0.84 (0.60–1.18)	0.88 (0.62–1.25)	0.11
Cellulose (g/day)	3.40	4.40	5.30	6.20	8.00	
RR* (95% CI)	1.0	0.75 (0.55–1.03)	0.71 (0.52–0.97)	0.78 (0.57–1.06)	0.47 (0.33–0.66)	0.0002
Multivariate RR† (95% CI)	1.0	0.76 (0.56–1.05)	0.74 (0.54–1.01)	0.83 (0.61–1.14)	0.52 (0.36–0.75)	0.002
Lignin (g/day)	1.00	1.20	1.50	1.80	2.40	
RR* (95% CI)	1.0	0.82 (0.60–1.12)	0.87 (0.64–1.19)	0.65 (0.47-.090)	0.53 (0.38–0.76)	0.0002
Multivariate RR† (95% CI)	1.0	0.83 (0.61–1.14)	0.89 (0.65–1.21)	0.71 (0.51–1.00)	0.62 (0.43–0.89)	0. 01

*Adjusted for age and total energy. CI denotes confidence interval.

†Adjusted for age, physical activity, and energy-adjusted total fat.

Dietary fibre is often a mixture of soluble and insoluble fibre[35]. In our data, the insoluble component of fibre was strongly associated with a decreased risk of DD, and this association was particularly strong for cellulose. Insoluble fibre is the major dietary fibre fraction and, overall, fruits and vegetables tend to be higher in cellulose than does cereal[36,37]. This might partially explain the observed beneficial effect of fibre from fruits and vegetables in our study. Cellulose comprises approximately one-third or less of the total fibre in most foods except for legumes, in which it is about half[37]. In fruits and vegetables the cellulose represented an average of 30+% and >50% of the insoluble fraction, respectively[37].

Soluble fibre is metabolized by colonic bacteria to a greater extent than insoluble fibre, and hence has little effect on stool weight[35,36]. However, fermentable fibre (mainly from fruits and vegetables) can increase faecal output by stimulating microbial growth. As a result of the stimulation of bacterial growth, dietary fibre is degraded to short-chain fatty acids (SCFA) and other products, such as methane, hydrogen, and carbon dioxide. Luminal SCFA are now recognized as an important fuel source for the colon[38], particularly in the distal colon, which is the most common site for DD. However, some 60+% of ingested cellulose appears in human faeces[39], which indicates that insoluble fibre is fermented to some degree since SCFA are not abolished when the diet contains insoluble fibre such as cellulose or wheat bran[40]. In an animal study it was also observed that insoluble fibre may modify the proportion of SCFA that are produced[41].

Micronutrients versus dietary fibre

Fibre intake from its different dietary sources is correlated with consumption of several micronutrients that may also be associated with lower risk of DD. Indeed, several such nutrients (e.g. potassium, beta-carotene, vitamin C, and magnesium) were all inversely related to the risk of DD. However, these inverse associations were no longer significant when each of these nutrients and energy-adjusted dietary fibre were entered in a multivariate model with age, energy-adjusted total fat, and physical activity, while the inverse association of dietary fibre and DD was not appreciably altered. This suggests, that fibre is indeed the important dietary variable, and not other constituents (vitamins and/or minerals) present in dietary fibre-rich foods[27].

Red meat, total fat and specific dietary fats

An association of red meat with DD was reported in an earlier case–control study in Greece[19], and recently from a study in the Orient, where right-sided diverticulosis is the predominant presentation[42]. Little was known as to whether total fat and/or specific dietary fats are associated with reduced risk of DD.

In our prospective study, for energy-adjusted total fat intake, the relative risks for men in each of the upper quintiles were elevated compared to men in the lowest quintile (Table 4). After energy adjustment, saturated and monounsaturated fat were both positively associated with the risk of DD

Table 4 Relative risk of DD by quintiles of total fat and specific dietary fats (adapted from ref. 27)

	Quintile					
Fats	*1*	*2*	*3*	*4*	*5*	*p-Value for trend**
Total fat (median g/day)	47.0	60.0	70.0	76.0	82.0	
Cases	55	76	100	58	98	
RR† (95% CI)	1.0	1.27 (0.90–1.81)	1.57 (1.13–2.19)	1.25 (0.86–1.83)	1.71 (1.0–2.37)	0.005
Multivariate RR‡ (95% CI)	1.0	1.17 (0.82–1.67)	1.40 (1.0–1.98)	1.09 (0.74–1.60)	1.38 (0.96–1.96)	0.20
Animal fat (median g/day)	22.0	31.0	37.0	43.0	52.0	
Cases	60	88	80	83	74	
RR† (95% CI)	1.0	1.66 (1.20–2.03)	1.39 (0.99–1.94)	1.57 (1.13–2.19)	1.43 (1.02–2.01)	0.12
Multivariate RR‡ (95% CI)	1.0	1.50 (1.08–2.10)	1.20 (0.85–1.69)	1.27 (0.90–1.80)	1.08 (0.75–1.56)	0.80
Vegetable fat (median g/day)	18.0	25.0	30.0	35.0	43.0	
Cases	70	73	85	70	87	
RR† (95% CI)	1.0	1.06 (0.76–1.47)	1.28 (0.93–1.75)	1.06 (0.76–1.48)	1.28 (0.94–1.76)	0.13
Multivariate RR‡ (95% CI)	1.0	1.07 (0.77–1.49)	1.30 (0.94–1.79)	1.08 (0.77–1.51)	1.32 (0.96–1.81)	0.10
Saturated fatty acids (median g/day)	15.1	20.9	24.3	26.7	30.3	
Cases	59	82	82	80	82	
RR† (95% CI)	1.0	1.45 (1.04–2.02)	1.54 (1.10–2.15)	1.51 (1.08–2.13)	1.61 (1.16–2.25)	0.01
Multivariate RR‡ (95% CI)	1.0	1.30 (0.92–1.83)	1.34 (0.94–1.89)	1.27 (0.89–1.81)	1.22 (0.85–1.76)	0.47
Monounsaturated fatty acids (median g/day)	16.5	22.4	26.0	28.6	31.2	
Cases	61	73	86	79	86	
RR† (95% CI)	1.0	1.26 (0.90–1.77)	1.45 (1.04–2.01)	1.41 (1.01–1.97)	1.53 (1.10–2.11)	0.01
Multivariate RR‡ (95% CI)	1.0	1.15 (0.81–1.62)	1.29 (0.92–1.81)	1.19 (0.84–1.68)	1.24 (0.87–1.75)	0.26

Table 4 (continued)

Fats	*Quintile* 1	2	3	4	5	*p-Value for trend**
Polyunsaturated fatty acids (median g/day)	8.6	11.3	12.8	14.6	17.4	
Cases	73	79	66	79	88	
RR[†] (95% CI)	1.0	1.14 (0.83–1.57)	0.95 (0.68–1.32)	1.14 (0.83–1.57)	1.25 (0.92–1.71)	0.19
Multivariate RR[‡] (95% CI)	1.0	1.15 (0.83–1.58)	0.95 (0.68–1.32)	1.14 (0.83–1.58)	1.28 (0.94–1.76)	0.16
Omega-3 fatty acids (median g/day)	<0.1	0.1	0.2	0.3	0.5	
Cases	72	86	83	77	67	
RR[†] (95% CI)	1.0	1.08 (0.79–1.47)	1.17 (0.86–1.61)	0.92 (0.67–1.27)	0.86 (0.61–1.19)	0.20
Multivariate RR[‡] (95% CI)	1.0	1.11 (0.81–1.52)	1.25 (0.91–1.71)	1.02 (0.74–1.41)	0.97 (0.69–1.36)	0.38
Trans fatty acids (median g/day)	1.9	2.7	3.2	3.7	4.6	
Cases	62	64	106	76	77	
RR[†] (95% CI)	1.0	1.28 (0.90–1.81)	1.73 (1.27–2.35)	1.70 (1.22–2.37)	1.49 (1.06–2.09)	0.002
Multivariate RR[‡] (95% CI)	1.0	1.17 (0.82–1.67)	1.52 (1.10–2.10)	1.46 (1.03–2.07)	1.29 (0.91–1.84)	0.25

*Test for trend was calculated by using the median intake of nutrients in each quintile as a continuous variable in a multiple logistic regression.

[†]Adjusted for age and total energy.

[‡]Adjusted for age, energy-adjusted dietary fibre and physical activity. CI denotes confidence interval.

(Table 4). Positive associations were also seen with *trans* fatty acids and polyunsaturated fat, whereas a weak inverse association was seen for the omega-3 fatty acid intake. However, when we also adjusted for physical activity and dietary fibre, the associations with total fat and types of fat were substantially attenuated and no longer significant (Table 4). This attenuation was primarily due to the influence of dietary fibre and to a lesser extent to physical activity.

After adjusting for age, dietary fibre, physical activity, and total energy, intake of red meat was positively associated with the risk of DD; however, the association was non-linear and the trend not statistically significant (RR = 1.48, 95% CI 1.00–2.19 for the highest quintile, p-value for trend = 0.24). Little suggestion of an association was seen with combined intake of chicken and fish, and with dairy fat.

Using a multivariate model controlling for age, physical activity, and total energy, we examined the risk of DD among the subjects classified jointly according to their intake of total dietary fibre and total fat or red meat. For men in the highest quintile of total fat intake and the lowest quintile of total dietary fibre intake (as compared with those in the opposite extreme), the risk of DD was more than doubled (Figure 1). Similarly for those in the highest category of red meat and the lowest quintile of total dietary fibre intake, the risk was tripled (Figure 2). We further analyzed groups described in Figures 1 and 2 to characterize the dietary patterns of the extreme categories. In general there was about a three-fold difference in the median intake of the high dietary fibre/low total fat or red meat group compared to the low dietary fibre/high

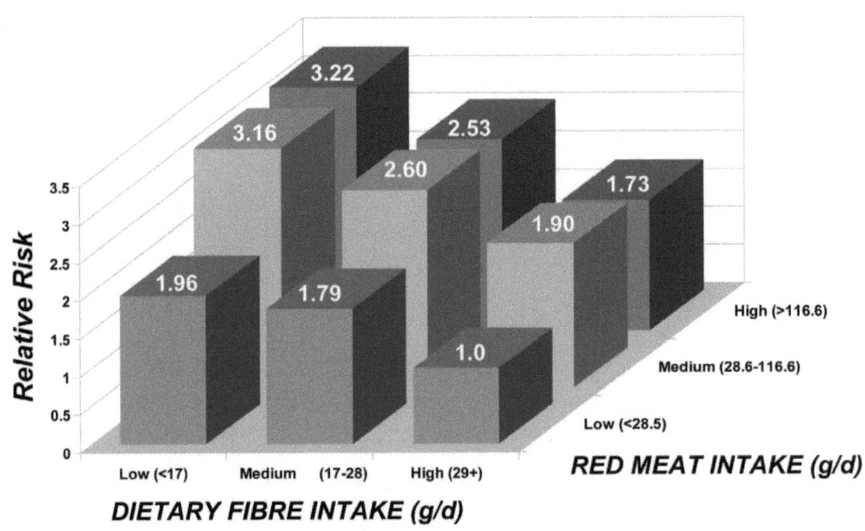

Figure 1 Relative risk (adjusted for age and total energy) of DD by levels of calorie-adjusted dietary fibre and red meat intake (adapted from ref. 27)

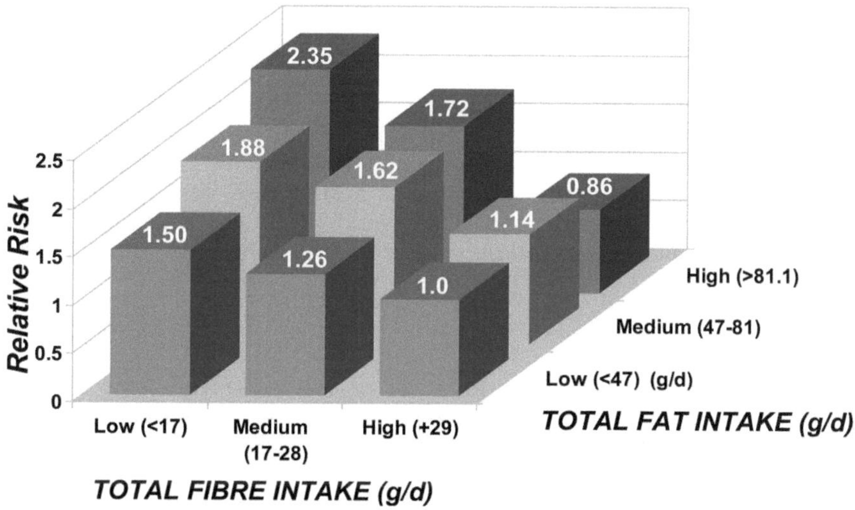

Figure 2 Relative risk (adjusted for age and total energy) of DD by levels of calorie-adjusted dietary fibre and total fat intake (adapted from ref. 27)

total fat or red meat group. Although differences were greater for total dietary fibre, rather than for any specific dietary fibre source, fruit fibre was the only fibre source which significantly discriminated between the high dietary fibre and the low dietary fibre group. Fruit fibre constituted about 33% of the total dietary fibre component in the high dietary fibre/low red meat or total fat group compared to about 10% in the low dietary fibre/high red meat or total fat group.

In our study the intake of chicken and fish meat was not appreciably associated with the risk of DD nor indeed was animal protein, which has not been shown to have any consistent effect on stool weight or transit time[43]. This supports the suggestion that, under the influence of red meat intake, bacteria may produce a 'toxic metabolite' or a spasmogen that weakens the wall of the colon and favours the formation of diverticula[44]. Whether red meat may influence DD by stimulating the release of bile acids through mechanisms unrelated to its fat or protein content, and whether there is a biological interaction between dietary fibre and red meat, needs to be explored. It was shown that patients with DD had a higher average daily faecal bile acid output than controls, which was reduced to near control levels after the administration of bran[45]. These changes led some to believe that DD is a motility disorder which may be reversed by a higher intake of dietary fibre[46]. The finding that red meat might be involved in the aetiology of DD may help to explain why vegetarians have a lower prevalence of diverticulosis than expected on the basis of their fibre intake[21].

Specific foods and the risk of DD

We also examined specific foods in relation to the risk of DD. Of the 131 foods included in the dietary questionnaire, 14 foods were significantly (p for trend $\leqslant 0.01$) associated with DD, either positively or inversely. These food items mainly discriminated between cases and non-cases, particularly for their crude and dietary fibre, total fat, and red meat intake. Among the strong positive associations were those with beef eaten as a main dish, and with processed meat[27]. Significant inverse trends for several fruits and vegetables largely account for the inverse associations of fruit and vegetable fibre with the risk of DD[27].

Alcohol

Several studies identified alcohol[47,48] as a risk factor for some digestive diseases. No association between alcohol and DD was reported in the only two case–control studies which addressed this relationship[19,49]; however, a prospective assessment has not been investigated. We examined the relationships of age-adjusted alcohol intake, and the separate effects of alcohol from beer, wine, and spirits with the risk of DD. Compared to non-drinkers, drinkers of more than 30 g of alcohol per day (two or three drinks/day) had an elevated risk of DD (Table 5). This association was attenuated in the multivariate analysis, and the trend was not statistically significant in either the age-adjusted or the multivariate analysis (Table 5). We also examined the separate effects of alcohol from beer, wine, and spirits in relation to the risk of DD. Intake of beer and wine (red and white) was not associated with the risk of DD (p for trend = 0.50 for beer, p for trend = 0.60 for wine), while intake of spirits was positively associated with the risk of DD (p for trend = 0.05). This positive association was nonlinear, and was evident among any level of spirits intake compared to never-drinkers[28].

We explored the possibility that the association between alcohol intake and DD was distorted, because our non-drinker category might have included some past heavy drinkers, current drinkers who denied drinking, or men who abstained because of illness. We therefore excluded 6230 men who reported on our 1986 semiquantitative food-frequency questionnaire a decrease in their drinking in the past 10 years, and who did not drink in 1986 (past drinkers). The relative risks were almost identical to that of the whole cohort (RR = 1.37, 95% CI 0.88–2.14 compared to the RR = 1.36, 95% CI 0.94–1.97 for the whole cohort). The association between alcohol and risk of DD was not modified appreciably by age when those who were under 65 years of age and 65 years and over were examined separately[28]. Our data suggest that moderate alcohol intake was not associated with an appreciable increased risk of DD. Because of the limited number of heavy drinkers in this study we could not address whether higher levels of alcohol consumption (50 g or more per day) might increase the risk. Misclassification is unlikely to have influenced our reported association appreciably since the dietary questionnaire reliably measures alcohol intake[50]. This slight, if any, increase in risk of DD is in sharp contrast to the much stronger association between alcohol and colorectal adenoma and cancer reported in this cohort[47].

Table 5 Relative risk of DD according to alcohol intake (adapted from ref. 28)

			Relative risk (95% CI)	
Alcohol	*Person-years*	*Observed cases*	*Age-adjusted*	*Multivariate**
None	44 265	77	Reference	Reference
0.1–5.0 g/day	51 007	108	1.28 (0.95–1.71)	1.30 (0.96–1.76)
5.1–10.0 g/day	31 323	62	1.20 (0.86–1.67)	1.38 (0.98–1.95)
10.1–15 g/day	20 756	39	1.09 (0.74–1.60)	1.13 (0.77–1.66)
15.1–30.0 g/day	25 751	58	1.28 (0.92–1.80)	1.16 (0.81–1.66)
30.1+	14 336	38	1.40 (0.95–2.07)	1.36 (0.94–1.97)
			(*p*-value for trend† = 0.15)	(*p*-value for trend† = 0.37)

*Adjusted for age, energy-adjusted dietary fibre and energy-adjusted total fat. CI denotes confidence interval.

†Test for trend was calculated by using the median alcohol intake in each category as continuous in a multiple logistic regression.

Caffeine

There are comparatively few epidemiological studies investigating the relationship between caffeine and most colonic diseases[51]. To our knowledge the association between caffeine, caffeine-containing beverages, and risk of DD has not been investigated. We observed a weak positive association between caffeine consumption and the risk of DD in the age-adjusted analysis; however, this association was attenuated in the multivariate model which also included physical activity, energy-adjusted intake of dietary fibre and total fat (Table 6). We also examined the relationship of coffee, tea, and decaffeinated coffee with the risk of DD. We observed little association between these beverages and the risk of DD comparing those who drank four or more cups per day to never-drinkers (Table 6). In this study we observed that risk of DD was not elevated in men who consumed large amounts of caffeine compared with those men who drank little or none. Similar findings were evident among different caffeine sources, mainly coffee and tea, and among men who consumed large amount of decaffeinated coffee. Our findings suggest that higher levels of caffeine do not appreciably increase the risk of DD.

NON-DIETARY FACTORS AND THE RISK OF DD

Physical activity

A limited number of studies have addressed the effect of physical activity on the colon, despite the widely held belief of a beneficial effect of exercise on gastrointestinal functions. A reduction in transit time was the consistent finding in most of the studies addressing the effect of exercise on colonic functions[52–55], although some did not observe such an effect[56]. An increase in colonic motor activity has also been postulated; however, the exact mechanism of this effect is still not clear. Some authors have suggested that the effect might be multifactorial, involving hormonal, vascular, and mechanical aspects[52]. The association of physical activity with the risk of DD, however, has not been prospectively investigated.

We examined the relationships of age-adjusted total physical activity, vigorous activity, and non-vigorous activity with the risk of DD. Total physical activity was inversely associated with the risk of DD. Compared to men in the lowest quintile of physical activity, those in the highest quintile had reduced their risk of DD by 43% (Table 7). Nearly all of this inverse association was attributable to the vigorous activities (Table 7). In contrast non-vigorous activity was not appreciably associated with risk of DD (Table 7). When we analysed separately total physical activity, vigorous activity and non-vigorous activity in multivariate models with age, energy-adjusted dietary fibre, and energy-adjusted total fat, our findings did not change appreciably from those in the age-adjusted model (Table 7).

Using a multivariate model controlling for age- and energy-adjusted total fat, we examined the risk of DD among the subjects classified jointly according to their intake of dietary fibre, and physical activity level. For men in the lowest

Table 6 Relative risk of DD by levels of total caffeine, coffee, tea, and decaffeinated coffee (adapted from ref. 28)

			Relative risk (95% CI)	
Variable	*Person-years*	*Observed cases**	*Age-adjusted*	*Multivariate*†
Caffeine (median mg/day)				
6.0	37 594	61	Reference	Reference
82	37 486	88	1.14 (1.01–1.94)	1.34 (0.97–1.86)
165	37 185	76	1.23 (0.88–1.71)	1.14 (0.81–1.61)
355	37 839	84	1.37 (0.98–1.90)	1.26 (0.91–1.77)
615	37 388	73	1.23 (0.87–1.73)	1.11 (0.78–1.57)
			(*p*-value for trend‡ = 0.25)	(*p*-value for trend‡ = 0.98)
Coffee (cups)				
Almost never	54 696	104	Reference	Reference
1–3/month to 1/day	65 672	135	1.05 (0.81–1.35)	1.0 (0.78–1.30)
2–3/day	42 813	89	1.09 (0.82–1.45)	1.01 (0.76–1.34)
⩾4–5/day	19 890	39	1.09 (0.75–1.58)	0.95 (0.65–1.38)
			(*p*-value for trend‡ = 0.53)	(*p*-value for trend‡ = 0.81)
Tea (cups)				
Almost never	76 599	138	Reference	Reference
1–3/month to 1/day	65 672	181	1.11 (0.89–1.38)	1.14 (0.91–1.42)
2–3/day	42 813	32	1.53 (1.04–2.24)	1.53 (1.04–2.26)
⩾4–5/day	2718	5	1.04 (0.43–2.55)	1.04 (0.42–2.54)
			(*p*-value for trend‡ = 0.09)	(*p*-value for trend‡ = 0.12)
Decaffeinated coffee (cups)				
Almost never	84 692	133	Reference	Reference
1–3/month to 1/day	69 941	167	1.41 (1.12–1.76)	1.51 (1.20–1.90)
2–3/day	20 600	53	1.45 (1.00–1.95)	1.56 (1.13–2.15)
⩾4–5/day	6456	12	1.08 (0.60–1.95)	1.12 (0.62–2.02)
			(*p*-value for trend‡ = 0.02)	(*p*-value for trend‡ = 0.17)

*Number of cases do not always add up to 382, because of missing information for specific beverages.

†Adjusted for age, energy-adjusted dietary fibre and energy-adjusted total fat.

‡Test for trend was calculated by using the median intake specific beverages in each category as continuous in a multiple logistic regression. CI denotes confidence interval.

Table 7 Relative risk of DD by physical activity, non-vigorous, and vigorous activity levels (adapted from ref. 29)

	Category					
Variable	*1*	*2*	*3*	*4*	*5*	*p-Value for trend*†
Total physical activity (median of total MET)¶	0.9	4.8	11.3	22.6	46.8	
RR* (95% CI)	1.0	0.89 (0.67–1.18)	0.67 (0.49–0.91)	0.68 (0.50–0.92)	0.57 (0.41–0.79)	0.0002
Multivariate RR‡ (95% CI)	1.0	0.91 (0.68–1.21)	0.71 (0.52–0.97)	0.74 (0.54–1.01)	0.63 (0.45–0.88)	0.008
Non-vigorous activity (median of total MET)§	0.1	1.4	3.4	7.6	20.8	
RR* (95% CI)	1.0	1.13 (0.83–1.55)	0.78 (0.56–1.10)	1.06 (0.77–1.46)	0.93 (0.67–1.30)	0.41
Multivariate RR‡ (95% CI)	1.0	1.15 (0.84–1.58)	0.79 (0.56–1.12)	1.09 (0.79–1.49)	0.93 (0.67–1.69)	0.65
Vigorous activity (median of total MET)††	0	3.5	15.0	41.0		
RR* (95% CI)	1.0	0.74 (0.57–0.97)	0.79 (0.61–1.03)	0.53 (0.37–0.75)		0.001
Multivariate RR‡ (95% CI)	1.0	0.78 (0.60–1.02)	0.88 (0.67–1.15)	0.60 (0.41–0.87)		0.01

*Adjusted for age.

†Test for trend was calculated by using the median total MET value of exercise in each category as a continuous variable in a multiple logistic regression. ‡Adjusted for age, energy-adjusted dietary fibre and energy-adjusted total fat. CI denotes confidence interval.

§Included flight of stairs climbed and walking or hiking outdoors (including walking at golf).

††Included running (10 min/mile or faster), jogging (slower than 10 min/mile), lap swimming, tennis, squash or racquetball, calisthenics or rowing, bicycling (including stationary machines).

¶Total MET = sum of the average time/week spent in each activity × MET value of each activity.

$$\text{MET value} = \frac{\text{caloric need/kg body weight/h during activity}}{\text{caloric need/kg body weight/h at rest}}$$

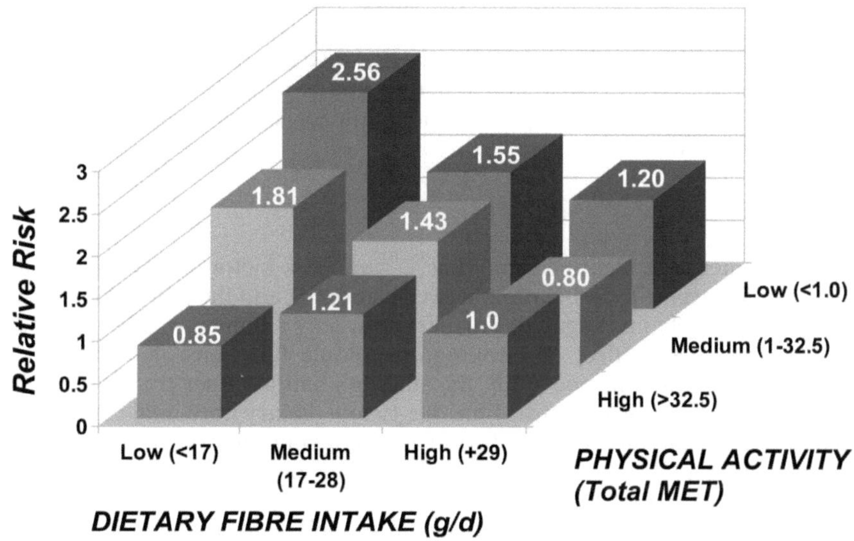

Figure 3 Relative risk (adjusted for age and total energy) of DD by levels of calorie-adjusted dietary fibre and physical activity

quintile for both dietary fibre and physical activity (as compared with those in the opposite extreme), the relative risk of DD was 2.56, 95% CI 1.36–4.82 (Figure 3). The association between low level of physical activity and risk of DD was strongest among men with low intake of fibre.

Whether physical activity may influence DD through any of the above-mentioned mechanisms or other mechanisms, and whether specific exercise (e. g. jogging and running) has specific effects on colonic functions needs to be explored[55].

Our findings suggest that increasing levels of physical activity reduce the risk of DD. They also provide evidence that the combination of low physical activity and a diet low in fibre particularly augments the risk.

Body mass index (BMI)

Obesity increases the risk of several diseases. Therefore, we investigated whether there is an association between high BMI and DD. Indeed, we observed a positive association between age-adjusted BMI and the risk of DD, however, this association was attenuated and not statistically significant, when we adjusted in multivariate models for other factors which also included physical activity, energy-adjusted dietary fibre, and energy-adjusted total fat[29]. Incidentally, age-adjusted total energy intake and height were not significantly associated with risk of DD[29]. Our data suggest that increasing BMI is not associated with any substantially increased risk of DD. However, a study reported that more severe DD was observed among young (<40 years) obese men[57]. We could not address this hypothesis, since the participants in our study are all over the age of 40 years. Whether age is a modifying factor for the severity of the symptomatic presentations and/or complications needs to be explored in future studies.

Smoking

Several studies have identified smoking[58–61] as a risk factor for several digestive diseases; however, the association between smoking and the risk of DD has not been prospectively investigated. Furthermore, only a limited number of studies have addressed the effect of smoking on colonic functions, in particular on colonic transit time. In one study the smokers had a longer transit time than non-smokers[62]. A longer transit time due to low dietary fibre intake can lead to increased intraluminal pressure, favouring the formation of diverticula[2].

When adjusted only for age, smoking was positively and significantly associated with risk of DD; however, this association was attenuated, and not significant, when assessed in multivariate models with age, physical activity, energy-adjusted intake of dietary fibre and total fat (Table 8). This attenuation was primarily due to the influence of dietary fibre, and to a lesser extent to physical activity. Overall, past smokers were not at increased risk compared to never-smokers. In a multivariate model with age, physical activity, energy-adjusted dietary fibre and energy-adjusted total fat, we examined the effect of time since quitting among past smokers compared to current smokers. We observed that the relative risk of current smoking was unchanged, and that the relative risks for having quit for 10 years or less and more than 10 years (compared to current smokers) were 0.94 (95% CI 0.64–1.39) and 0.88 (95% CI 0.69–1.13), respectively. In our overall data we did not find a substantial positive association between smoking and DD. Smokers in the highest category (40 pack-years) had a 21% greater risk of DD than never-smokers[28]. When we assessed current smokers by number of cigarettes smoked daily, an almost similar increased risk (25%) was noted. The risk among past smokers was not elevated among men who stopped smoking 3 or more years prior to the diagnosis of DD.

Our findings indicate that some independent association with smoking may exist, but any effect does not seem to be large. In contrast to findings for DD, we found a strong positive association between smoking and risk of colorectal adenoma and cancer in this cohort[60].

Anti-inflammatory and analgesic use and the risk of DD

Considering that the majority of DD cases are asymptomatic, it is important to study the possible factors that might determine the development and severity of the symptomatic presentation of this disease, which are not well understood. Several reports have suggested an association between consumption of steroids, non-steroidal anti-inflammatory drugs (NSAID), and the complications of DD[63–67]. NSAID are among the most widely used

Table 8 Relative risk of DD by smoking status (adapted from ref. 28)

Variable	*Person-years*	*Observed cases**	*Relative risk (95% CI)*	
			Age-adjusted	*Multivariate*†
Smoking status				
Non-smokers	84 506	159	Reference	Reference
Past smokers	77 912	163	0.98 (0.79–1.22)	0.96 (0.77–1.19)
Current smokers (cig/day)				
1–14 cig/day	4820	10	1.03 (0.55–1.96)	0.94 (0.50–1.80)
15–24 cig/day	5810	18	1.52 (0.93–2.47)	1.28 (0.78–2.11)
25+ cig/day	5347	17	1.55 (0.94–2.55)	1.25 (0.75–2.09)
			(*p*-value for trend‡ = 0.05)	(*p*-value for trend‡ = 0.36)

*Numbers of cases do not always add up to 382, because of missing information for smoking.

†Adjusted for age, energy-adjusted dietary fibre, and energy-adjusted total fat. CI denotes confidence interval

‡Test for trend is calculated by using the median number of cigarettes smoked across categories of current smoking in a multiple logistic regression.

medications in the world. Because their use is particularly frequent among the elderly, and DD is common in this age group, even modest changes in the risk of side-effects may have important public health implications. It is known that aspirin and NSAID might have a deleterious effect on the upper gastrointestinal tract[68–71]; however, only recently have these medications been suggested to be potentially harmful to the lower gastrointestinal tract[72]. Little information exists concerning adverse effects on the lower gastrointestinal tract, if any, for regular use of either aspirin and acetaminophen. Most studies of medication use in relation to DD have also been limited by the number of subjects, failure to adjust for potential risk factors such as dietary fibre, other dietary and non-dietary factors such as physical activity, and the possibility of recall and selection bias in case–control studies. Therefore, we examined prospectively the relationship between self-reported regular use of NSAID, acetaminophen, oral steroids, and aspirin and the risk of symptomatic DD[31].

We observed an overall increased risk for symptomatic DD among regular NSAID and acetaminophen users compared to non-users (Table 9). The positive association between NSAID and acetaminophen use and the risk of symptomatic DD became stronger with evidence of more consistent use of

Table 9 Relative risk of DD by NSAID and acetaminophen use in the HPFS (adapted from ref. 31)

Variable	*NSAID and acetaminophen use*	
	1988	*1988 + 1990*
Follow-up period	*1988 to 1992*	*1990 to 1992*
NSAID[§]		
Non-users, cases/person-years	265/122 249	118/51 475
Users, cases/person-years*	45/13 682	34/8745
Age-adjusted RR (95% CI)[†]	1.52 (1.11–2.08)	2.19 (1.28–3.76)
Multivariate RR (95% CI)[‡]	1.50 (1.09–2.06)	2.24 (1.28–3.91)
p-Value	0.01	0.004
Acetaminophen		
Non-users, cases/person-years	286/128 091	133/55 314
Users, cases/person-years*	24/7840	19/4906
Age-adjusted RR (95% CI)[†]	1.40 (0.93–2.13)	1.82 (0.81–4.07)
Multivariate RR (95% CI)[‡]	1.33 (0.88–2.03)	1.81 (0.79–4.11)
p-Value	0.18	0.16

*Participants who reported NSAID and acetaminophen use (the follow-up period for1988 was 1988–1992; for 1988 and 1990, 1990–1992); non-users reported no NSAID or acetaminophen use during the specified time periods. †Age-adjusted relative risk and 95% CI for users compared with non-users of NSAID or acetaminophen for each of the specified time periods. ‡Relative risk adjusted for age, physical activity, energy-adjusted dietary fibre and total fat. §Does not include aspirin. NSAID indicates non-steroidal anti-inflammatory drug.

both medications; that is, regular use of both medications reported on both the 1988 and 1990 questionnaires. The relative risk did not change appreciably when we controlled for risk factors, physical activity, and energy-adjusted dietary fibre and total fat (all in quintiles) (Table 9).

We further explored the association between NSAID and acetaminophen use and the risk of DD by specific presenting symptoms. We observed an increased risk of DD among cases whose symptoms were mainly abdominal pain and change in bowel habits, particularly with evidence of more consistent use of NSAID (Table 10). We also observed an increased risk of symptomatic DD with regular and consistent use of NSAID and acetaminophen, among the patients whose presenting symptoms were mainly bleeding. This positive association was substantial, particularly among regular and consistent acetaminophen users (Table 11). The positive association of acetaminophen was further strengthened when we excluded from our analysis participants with known upper gastrointestinal tract conditions associated with bleeding (such as gastric or duodenal ulcers), or with a history of liver diseases (RR for acetaminophen = 18.65, 95% CI 4.63–75.10). Moreover, when we considered the cases diagnosed in the last 2 years of our follow-up who reported regular acetaminophen use on the 1986 baseline questionnaire, and also on the consecutive follow-up questionnaires in 1988 and 1990, the positive association of acetaminophen with the risk of bleeding diverticula was further increased (RR = 27.30, 95% CI 11.42–65.24). However, the risk of symptomatic presentation of diverticula in general, and of bleeding in

Table 10 Relative risk of DD for participants whose main symptoms were abdominal pain and change in bowel habits, by NSAID and acetaminophen use in the HPFS (adapted from ref. 31)

Variable	*NSAID and acetaminophen use*	
Follow-up period	*1988* *1988 to 1992*	*1988 + 1990* *1990 to 1992*
NSAID[§]		
Non-users, cases/person-years	200/122 249	89/51 475
Users, cases/person-years*	30/13 682	24/8745
Age-adjusted RR (95% CI)[†]	1.35 (0.92–1.98)	2.27 (1.24–4.17)
Multivariate RR (95% CI)[‡]	1.33 (0.91–1.96)	2.32 (1.24–4.35)
p-Value	0.14	0.009
Acetaminophen		
Non-users, cases/person-years	216/128 091	102/55 314
Users, cases/person-years*	14/7840	11/4906
Age-adjusted RR (95% CI)[†]	1.09 (0.63–1.87)	1.17 (0.37–3.69)
Multivariate RR (95% CI)[‡]	1.04 (0.60–1.79)	1.18 (0.37–3.71)
p-Value	0.89	0.78

*Participants who reported NSAID and acetaminophen use (the follow-up period for1988 was 1988–1992; for 1988 and 1990, 1990–1992); non-users reported no NSAID or acetaminophen use during the specified time periods. [†]Age-adjusted relative risk and 95% CI for users compared with non-users of NSAID or acetaminophen for each of the specified time periods. [‡]Relative risk adjusted for age, physical activity, energy-adjusted dietary fibre and total fat. [§]Does not include aspirin. NSAID indicates non-steroidal anti-inflammatory drug.

Table 11 Relative risk of DD for participants whose main symptoms were bleeding, by NSAID and acetaminophen use in the HPFS (adapted from ref. 31)

Variable	*NSAID and acetaminophen use*	
	1988	*1988 + 1990*
Follow-up period	*1988 to 1992*	*1990 to 1992*
NSAID[§]		
Non-users, cases/person-years	28/122 249	9/51 475
Users, cases/person-years*	7/13 682	5/ 8745
Age-adjusted RR (95% CI)[†]	2.23 (0.99–4.99)	4.20 (1.03–17.17)
Multivariate RR (95% CI)[‡]	2.15 (0.94–4.93)	4.64 (0.99–21.74)
p-Value	0.07	0.05
Acetaminophen		
Non-users, cases/person-years	28/128 091	8/55 314
Users, cases/person-years*	7/7840	6/4906
Age-adjusted RR (95% CI)[†]	4.11 (1.93–8.77)	14.62 (5.38–39.71)
Multivariate RR (95% CI)[‡]	3.75 (1.63–8.64)	13.63 (3.53–52.6)
p-Value	0.002	0.0002

*Participants who reported NSAID and acetaminophen use (the follow-up period for1988 was 1988–1992; for 1988 and 1990, 1990–1992); non-users reported no NSAID or acetaminophen use during the specified time periods. †Age-adjusted relative risk and 95% CI for users compared with non-users of NSAID or acetaminophen for each of the specified time periods. ‡Relative risk adjusted for age, physical activity, energy-adjusted dietary fibre and total fat. §Does not include aspirin. NSAID indicates non-steroidal anti-inflammatory drug.

particular, was not as substantially elevated for NSAID users who reported regular intake on only one of the follow-up questionnaires, and who were diagnosed within the corresponding 2-year follow-up period (RR of bleeding for self-reported use of NSAID on the 1988 or 1990 questionnaires = 1.48, 95% CI 0.44–4.99 and RR = 2.81, 95% CI 0.83–9.48 respectively; RR for bleeding for acetaminophen use = 1.73, 95% CI 0.42–7.18 and RR = 8.48, 95% CI 3.21–22.43 respectively). The association between NSAID and acetaminophen use and the risk of bleeding was higher among regular and consistent users who were under the age of 65 years, than those who were over 65 years of age (for users under the age of 65 years, RR for NSAID = 6.00, 95% CI 1.22–29.46; RR for acetaminophen = 9.90, 95% CI 1.98–49.37).

We did not observe any increase in the risk of symptomatic DD among regular and consistent aspirin users (for overall symptoms RR = 0.80, 95% CI 0.55–1.18; RR for abdominal pain and change in bowel habits = 0.78, 95% CI 0.50–1.21; RR for faecal occult blood = 1.29, 95% CI 0.47–3.48; RR for bleeding = 0.60, 95% CI 0.12–2.93). This association was generally similar between men under or over the age of 65 years. We observed an elevated risk of symptomatic DD among patients who reported regular and consistent use of oral corticosteroid, particularly among the cases who presented with abdominal pain and change in bowel habits. However, too few men among this cohort were taking oral corticosteroid consistently to provide stable estimates (RR for abdominal pain and change in bowel habits = 2.16, 95% CI 0.29–11.53).

The findings for NSAID use, and the risk of bleeding of diverticula in our study, concur with the findings of other reports[63–67]. Our findings could have arisen if the symptoms (such as bleeding),were related to an underlying condition for which NSAID were used. This possibility is unlikely, because we have eliminated many conditions which might be associated with abdominal symptoms (such as pain or bleeding) and, in view of their known effects on the stomach and duodenum, it is unlikely that NSAID would be used for abdominal symptoms. Rather they are the most widely used agents to treat musculoskeletal and arthritic conditions[73], which are not generally known to be associated with such symptoms. Most NSAID inhibit the action of prostaglandin synthetase[74], which is believed to be responsible for some of these complications, since prostaglandin may exert a gastrointestinal cytoprotective effect that is abolished by these medications[63,65,75–77]. This inhibition of prostaglandin effects by NSAID might impair the ability of the colon to limit inflammatory processes occurring within diverticula; they might also inhibit platelet aggregation[66,78] so that bleeding might occur in the presence of a bowel lesion (such as a diverticula). Alternatively, or in addition, they may mask symptoms so that patients present with more advanced disease[65,66]. However, the effect of NSAID could be unrelated to their influence on prostaglandin synthetase, and could exert a direct cytolytic action on the gut mucosa, as in the case with fenmates which are associated with mild colitis[79,80], and other NSAID that can occasionally cause ulcerative proctitis or colitis[81]. Furthermore, animal studies indicate that NSAID-induced intestinal lesions could be influenced by intestinal flora[82], food[83], and the enterohepatic circulation[84].

In our study the regular and consistent use of acetaminophen was associated with an elevated risk of bleeding of diverticula, and this risk remained elevated even when we adjusted for the use of other medications. This finding was unexpected, since acetaminophen is often considered as an attractive alternative analgesic to many NSAID indications, because of their potential gastrointestinal side-effects[71]. Acetaminophen toxicity related to the kidneys and the liver, particularly with alcohol intake, have been reported[85,86], but in most studies of upper gastrointestinal toxicity of acetaminophen no association has been found, although some adverse effects have been reported[87,88]. Epidemiological studies of potential adverse effect of regular and consistent use of acetaminophen on the lower gastrointestinal tract are few. However, in one study acetaminophen ingestion was reported to be associated with relapse in patients with ulcerative colitis[89]. Acetaminophen is generally considered to be a weak inhibitor of cyclooxygenase, and its effect on the metabolism of arachidonic acid is tissue-dependent. Potentially, acetaminophen can induce prostaglandin deficiency, which could lead to ulceration due to the loss of mucosal protection and bleeding due to platelet defective function[89–91].

Our study differed from previous reports by the availability of information about potentially confounding factors, such as dietary factors, alcohol intake, BMI, and physical activity which were assessed and updated at different follow-up periods and controlled for. The use of NSAID, acetaminophen, and other related medications which might cause similar adverse effect (such as steroids), was also assessed at several times throughout the study; furthermore, two separate assessments of NSAID and acetaminophen use allowed comparisons of long-term consistent users and non-users. Finally, the relatively homogeneous background of participants in the health professionals increases the likelihood of accurate exposure and outcome reporting, and decreases the likelihood of residual confounding.

Addressing bias and diverticular disease diagnosis in the HPFS

Biased recall of the dietary and non-dietary information was unlikely because the data were collected before the diagnosis of DD. We recognize that, as in almost every study, some degree of misclassification is inevitable. However, the prospective design of this study means that any misclassification would be random with regard to case status, and hence would tend to attenuate any association. Considering that the majority of DD cases are asymptomatic, and that diagnosis is made when affected individuals develop symptoms, we explored the possibility that the associations we observed were due to detection bias which might be related to their level of dietary fibre intake or physical activity level. For example, people with low dietary fibre intake, or who are not physically active, might have more abdominal symptoms, and hence more endoscopies, in which diverticulosis is diagnosed. However, the opposite was found; that is those participants in the HPFS who reported having endoscopies for abdominal symptoms were in fact eating more dietary fibre, less total fat, and were more physically active. We therefore conclude that detection bias is unlikely to have appreciably influenced our results.

Gaps in our knowledge about DD

Although our findings are most directly generalizable to non-vegetarian men 40 years and older, future studies should explore whether age is a modifying factor for the severity of the symptomatic presentations and/or complications. Although our prospective study was conducted among men, we have no reason to believe that the association we observed in men would be different for women, considering that there are no differences in the prevalence of the disease by gender. However, future studies should explore any possible differences in the relations between dietary and non-dietary factors, and the occurrence of DD due to gender. Considering that the majority of DD cases are asymptomatic, we still need to understand the mechanism of why the diverticula become symptomatic. We further need to assess whether specific factors are important for the formation of diverticula, and whether different factors contribute to the symptomatic presentation and/or complications. In summary, there are still many gaps in our understanding of the potential interactions between colonic structure, motility, diet, lifestyle, genetic factors and ethnicity (right-sided predominance in the Orient) and the aetiology of DD and its complications.

Can we prevent DD?

These prospective data support the hypothesis that high intake of dietary fibre mainly from fruits and vegetables reduces the risk of DD. The insoluble component of fibre was strongly associated with a decreased risk of DD, and this association was particularly strong for cellulose. Our findings also suggest that increasing levels of physical activity reduce the risk of DD. Risks were particularly elevated among men with the combination of high intake of total fat or red meat, low physical activity and low consumption of dietary fibre. There was an indication that some independent association with smoking and increasing BMI may exist, but any effect does not seem to be large. Moderate alcohol intake is not associated with an appreciable increased risk of DD.

These prospective data suggest that regular and consistent use of NSAID and acetaminophen is associated with symptoms of complicated DD, such as bleeding, particularly with acetaminophen use.

In summary, the strongest evidence so far suggests that physical activity, along with a high fibre diet, may be an important factor in the prevention of DD.

Acknowledgements

I am indebted to the participants in the Health Professionals Follow-up Study for making this study possible; to my colleagues Drs Walter Willett, Edward Giovannucci, Eric Rimm, Dimitrious Trichopoulos, Meir Stampfer, Graham Colditz, and Alberto Ascherio, for their guidance and insight; and to Alvin Wing, Helene Rockett, Laura Sampson, Jill Arnold, Elizabeth Frost-Hawes, Mildred Wolff, Cindy Dyer, Jan Vomacka, Kerry Pillsworth, and Mira Koyfman for their expert help.

References

1. Walters DAK, Smith AN. Strength of the colon wall in diverticular disease. Br J Surg. 1990; 77:257–9.
2. Painter NS, Burkitt DP. Diverticular disease of the colon: a deficiency disease of western civilization. Br Med J. 1971;2:450–4.
3. Parks TG. Natural history of diverticular disease of the colon. Clin Gastroenterol. 1975;4: 53–68.
4. Painter NS, Burkitt DP. Diverticular disease of the colon: a 20th century problem. Clin Gastroenterol. 1975;4:3–21.
5. Stollman N, Raskin JB. Diverticular disease of the colon. Lancet. 2004;363:631–9.
6. Parks TG. Natural history of diverticular disease of the colon;a review of 521 Cases. Br Med J. 1969;4:639–45.
7. Levien DH, Mazier WP, Surrell JA, Raiman PJ. Safe resection for diverticular disease of the colon. Dis Colon Rectum. 1989;32:30–2.
8. Munson KD, Hensien MA, Jacob LN, Robinson AM, Liston WA. Diverticulitis: a comprehensive follow-up. Dis Colon Rectum. 1996;39:318–22.
9. Wedell J, Banzhaf G, Chaoui R, Fischer R, Reichmann J. Surgical management of complicated colonic diverticulitis. Br J Surg. 1997;84:380–3.
10. Roberts PL, Veidenheimer MC. Diverticular disease of the colon. In: Bayless TM, editor. Current Therapy in Gastroenterology and Liver Diseases, 3rd edn. Toronto: Decker, 1990: 416–19.
11. Thompson WG, Patel DG. Clinical picture of diverticular disease of the colon. Clin Gastroenterol. 1986;15:903–16.
12. Sandler RS, Everhart JE, Donowitz M et al. The burden of selected digestive diseases in the United States. Gastroenterology. 2002;122:1500–11.

13. Painter N. Diverticular disease of the colon. In: Trowell H, Burkitt D, Heaton K, editors. Dietary Fibre, Fibre-depleted Foods and Diseases. London: Academic Press, 1985:145–60.
14. Lee YS. Diverticular disease of the large bowel in Singapore: an autopsy study. Dis Colon Rectum. 1986;29:330–5.
15. Levy N, Stermer E, Simon J. The changing epidemiology of diverticular disease in Israel. Dis Colon Rectum. 1985;28:416–18.
16. Ogunbiyi OA. Diverticular disease of the colon in Ibadan, Nigeria. Afr J Med Sci. 1989;18: 241–4.
17. Brodribb AJM, Humphreys DM. Diverticular disease: three studies. I. Relation to other disorders and fibre intake. Br Med J. 1976;1:424–5.
18. Leaky AL, Ellis RM, Quill DS, Peel ALG. High fibre diet in symptomatic diverticular disease of the colon. Ann R Coll Surg Engl. 1985;67:173–4.
19. Manousos O, Day NE, Tzonou A et al. Diet and other factors in the aetiology of diverticulosis: an epidemiological study in Greece. Gut. 1985;26:544–9.
20. Miettinen TA, Tarpila S. Fecal beta-sitosterol in patients with diverticular disease of the colon and in vegetarians. Scand J Gastroenterol. 1978;13:573–6.
21. Gear JSS, Ware A, Fursdon P et al. Symptomless diverticular disease and intake of dietary fiber. Lancet. 1979;1:511–14.
22. Findlay JM, Smith AN, Mitchell WD, Anderson AJB, Eastwood MA. Effects of unprocessed bran on colon function in normal subjects and in diverticular disease. Lancet. 1974;1:146–9.
23. Hodgson WJB. An interim report on the production of colonic diverticula in the rabbit. Gut. 1972;13:802–4.
24. Fisher N, Berry CS, Fearn T, Gregory JA, Hardy J. Cereal dietary fiber consumption and diverticular disease: a lifespan study in rats. Am J Clin Nutr. 1985;42:788–804.
25. Jaskiewicz K, Rossouw JE, Kritchevsky D, Van Resburg SJ, Fincham JE, Woodroof CW. The influence of diet and diemethylhydrazine on the small and large intestine of Vervet monkeys. Br J Exp Pathol. 1986;67:361–9.
26. Willett WC. Nutritional Epidemiology, 2nd edn. New York: Oxford University Press; 1998: 3–17.
27. Aldoori WH, Giovannucci EL, Rimm EB, Wing AL, Trichopoulos DV, Willett WC. A prospective study of diet and the risk of symptomatic diverticular disease in men. Am J Clin Nutr. 1994;60:757–64.
28. Aldoori WH, Giovannucci EL, Rimm EB, Wing AL, Trichopoulos DV, Willett WC. A prospective study of alcohol, smoking, caffeine, and the risk of symptomatic diverticular disease in men. Ann Epidemiol. 1995;5:221–8.
29. Aldoori WH, Giovannucci EL, Rimm EB et al. A prospective study of physical activity and the risk of symptomatic diverticular disease in men. Gut. 1995;36:276–82.
30. Aldoori WH, Giovannucci EL, Rockett HRH, Sampson L, Rimm EB, Willett WC. A prospective study of dietary fiber types and symptomatic diverticular disease in men. J Nutr. 1998;128:714–19.
31. Aldoori WH, Giovannucci EL, Rimm EB, Wing AL, Willett WC. Use of acetaminophen and nonsteroidal anti-inflammatory drugs. A prospective study and the risk of symptomatic diverticular disease in men. Arch Fam Med. 1998;7:255–60.
32. Klurfeld DM. The role of dietary fiber in gastrointestinal disease. J Am Diet Assoc. 1987; 87:1172–7.
33. Smith AN, Drummond E, Eastwood MA. The effect of coarse and fine Canadian red spring wheat and French soft wheat bran on colonic motility in patients with diverticular disease. Am J Clin Nutr. 1981;34:2460–3.
34. Heller SN, Hackler LR, Rivers JM et al. Dietary fiber: the effect of particle size of wheat bran on colonic funcion in young adult men. Am J Clin Nutr. 1980;33:1734–44.
35. Bennett WG, Creda JJ. Benefits of dietary fiber. Myth or Medicine? Postgrad Med. 1996;99: 153–75.
36. Slavin JL. Dietary fiber: classification, chemical analyses, and food sources. J Am Diet Assoc. 1987;87:1164–71.
37. Marlett JA. Content and composition of dietary fiber in 117 frequently consumed foods. J Am Diet Assoc. 1992;92:175–86.
38. Rabassa AA, Rogers AI. The role of short chain fatty acid metabolism in colonic disorders. Am J Gastroenterol. 1992;87:419–23.

39. Topping DL, Illman RJ. Bacterial fermentation in the human large bowel: time to change from the roughage model of dietary fibre? Med J Aust. 1986;144:307–9.
40. Topping DL. Soluble fiber polysaccharides: effects on plasma cholesterol and colonic fermentation. Nutr Rev. 1991;49:195–203.
41. Cheng BQ, Trimble RP, Illman RJ, Stone BA, Topping DL. Comparative effects of dietary wheat bran and its morphological components (aleurone and pericarp-seed coat) on volatile fatty acid concentrations in rat. Br J Nutr. 1987;57:69–76.
42. Lin OS, Soon MS, Wu SS, Chen YY, Hwang KL, Triadafilopoulos G. Dietary habits and right-sided colonic diverticulosis. Dis Colon Rectum. 2000;43:1412–18.
43. Cummings JH, Hill MJ, Bone ES, Branch WJ, Jenkins DJA. The effect of meat protein and dietary fiber on colonic function and metabolism. II. Bacterial metabolites in faeces and urine. Am J Clin Nutr. 1979;32:2094–101.
44. Heaton KW. Diet and diverticulosis: new leads. Gut. 1985;26:541–3.
45. Tarpila S, Miettinen TA, Metsaranta L. Effect of bran on serum cholesterol, faecal mass, fat bile acids and neutral sterols, and biliary lipids in patients with diverticular disease of the colon. Gut. 1978;19:137–45.
46. Eastwood MA, Walters DAK, Smith AN. Diverticular disease, is it a motility disorder? Clin Gastroenterol. 1982;11:545–61.
47. Giovannucci EL, Stampfer ML, Colditz GA. Folate, methionine, and alcohol intake and risk of colorectal adenoma. J Natl Cancer Inst. 1993;85:875–84.
48. Stemmerman GN, Nomura AM, Chyou PH, Yoshizawa C. Prospective study of alcohol intake and large bowel cancer. Dig Dis Sci. 1990;35:1414–20.
49. Manousos ON, Vrachliotis G, Papaevangelou G. Relation of diverticulosis of the colon to environmental factors in Greece. Dig Dis Sci. 1973;18:174–6.
50. Giovannucci EL, Colditz GA, Stampfer MJ. The assessment of alcohol consumption by a simple self-administered questionnaire. Am J Epidemiol. 1991;133:801–17.
51. Snowdon DA, Philips RL. Coffee consumption and risk of fatal cancers. Am J Public Health. 1984;74:820–3.
52. Oettle GJ. Effect of moderate exercise on bowel habit. Gut. 1991;32:941–4.
53. Koffler KH, Menkes A, Redmond RA, Whitehead WE, Pratley RE, Hurley BF. Strength training accelerates gastrointestinal transit in middle-aged and older men. Med Sci Sports Exerc. 1992;24:415–19.
54. Dapoigny M, Saran SK. Effects of physical exercise on colonic motor activity. Am J Physiol. 1990;260:G646–52.
55. Sullivan SN. The effect of running on gastrointestinal tract. J Clin Gastroenterol. 1984;6: 461–5.
56. Bingham SA, Cummings JH. Effect of exercise and physical fitness on large intestinal function. Gastroenterology. 1989;97:1389–99.
57. Dchauer PR, Ramos R, Ghiatas AA, Sirinek KR. Virulent diverticular disease in young obese men. Am J Surg. 1992;164:443–8.
58. Doll R, Peto R. Mortality in relation to smoking: 20 years' observation on male British doctors. Br Med J. 1976;2:1525–36.
59. Carsten JM, Pershagen G, Eklund G. Mortality in relation to cigarette and pipe smoking: 16 years' observation of 2500 Swedish men, J Epidemiol Community Health. 1987;41:166–72.
60. Giovannucci E, Rimm EB, Stampfer MJ et al. A prospective study of cigarette smoking and risk of colorectal adenoma and cancer in men, J Natl Cancer Inst. 1994;86:192–8.
61. Logan RFA, Somerville KW, Edmond M, Langman MJS. Is cigarette smoking associated with Crohn's disease? Gut. 1983;A980 (Abstract).
62. Meier R, Beglinger C, Dederding JP et al: Alters- und geschlechtsspezifische Normwerte der Dickdarmtransitzeit bei Gesunden. Scweiz Med Wochenschr. 1992;122:940–3.
63. Coutrot S, Roland D, Barbier J, Van Der Marcq P, Alcalay M, Matuchansky C. Acute perforation of colonic diverticula associated with short-term indomethacin. Lancet. 1978;2: 1055–6.
64. Langman MJS, Morgan L, Worrall A. Use of anti-inflammatory drugs by patients admitted with small or large bowel perforations and haemorrhage. Br Med J. 1985;290:347–9.
65. Corder A. Steroids, non-steroidal anti-inflammatory drugs, and serious septic complications of diverticular disease. Br Med J. 1987;295:1238.
66. Wilson RG, Smith AN, Macintyre IMC. Complications of diverticular disease and non-steroidal anti-inflammatory drugs: a prospective study. Br J Surg. 1990;77:1103–4.

67. Campbell K, Steele RJC. Non-steroidal anti-inflammatory drugs and complicated diverticular disease: a case–control study. Br J Surg. 1991;78:190–1.
68. Levy M. Aspirin use in patients with major upper gastrointestinal bleeding and peptic ulcer disease. N Engl J Med. 1974;290:1158–63.
69. Guess HA, West R, Strand LM et al. Fatal upper gastrointestinal hemorrhage or perforation among users and nonusers of nonsteroidal anti-inflammatory drugs in Saskatchewan, Canada 1983. J Clin Epidemiol. 1988;41:35–45.
70. Gabriel SE, Jaakkimainen L, Bombardier C. Risk for serious gastrointestinal complications related to use of nonsteroidal anti-inflammatory drugs. Ann Intern Med. 1991;115:787–96.
71. Willett LR, Carson JL, Storm BL. Epidemiology of gastrointestinal damage associated with nonsteroidal anti-inflammatory drugs. Drug Safety. 1994;10:170–81.
72. Rampton DS. Non-steroidal anti-inflammatory drugs and the lower gastrointestinal tract. Scand J Gastroenterol. 1987;22:1–4.
73. Baum C, Kennedy DL, Forbes MB. Utilization of nonsteroidal anti-inflammatory drugs. Arthritis Rheum. 1985;28:686–92.
74. Avron J. Reporting drug side effects: signals and noise (editorial). J Am Med Assoc. 1990; 263:1823.
75. Metz SA. Anti-inflammatory agents as inhibitors of prostaglandin synthesis in man. Med Clin N Am. 1981;65:713–57.
76. Kalmykov SV, Kazimorvskaia VB, Batunova EV. Rapid chemiluminescence analysis of the effects of drugs on functional activity of phagocytosing blood cells. Farmakol Toksikol. 1989;52:97–100.
77. Huy DP, Roch-Arvellier M, Lenoir M, Muntaner D, Thuret A, Giroud JP. *In-vitro* and *in-vivo* effects of piroxicam on rat polymorphonuclear responsiveness after induction of two acute non-specific inflammatory reactions. Agents Action. 1986;18:366–71.
78. Vane JR. The mode of action of aspirin and similar compounds. J Allergy Clin Immunol. 1976;58:691–712.
79. Gullikson GW, Sender M, Bass P. Laxative-like effects of nonsteroidal anti-inflammatory drugs on intestinal fluid movement and membrane integrity. J Pharmacol Exp Ther. 1982; 220:236–42.
80. Issacs PET, Sladen GE, Filpie I. Mefenamic acid enteropathy. J Clin Pathol. 1987;40:1221–7.
81. Ravi S, Keat AC, Keat ECB. Colitis caused by nonsteroidal anti-inflammatory drugs. Postgrad Med J. 1986;62:773–6.
82. Kent TH, Cardelli RM, Stamler FW. Small intestinal ulcers and intestinal flora in rats given indomethacin. Am J Pathol. 1969;53:237–49.
83. Satoh H, Guth PH, Grossman MI. Role of food in gastrointestinal ulceration produced by indomethacin in the rat. Gastroenterology. 1982;83:210–15.
84. Brodie DA, Cook PG, Bauer BJ, Dagie GE. Indomethacin-induced intestinal lesions in the rat. Toxicol Appl Pharmacol. 1970;17:615–24.
85. Rex DK, Kumar S. Recognizing acetaminophen hepatotoxicity in chronic alcoholics. Postgrad Med. 1992;91:241–5.
86. Bonkovsky HL, Kane RE, Jones DP, Galinsky RE, Barner B. Acute hepatic and renal toxicity from low doses of acetaminophen in the absence of alcohol abuse or malnutrition: evidence for increased susceptibility to drug toxicity due to cardiopulmonary and renal insufficiency. Hepatology. 1994;19:1141–8.
87. Savage RL, Moller PW, Ballantyre CL, Wells JE. Variation in the risk of peptic ulcer complications with nonsteroidal anti-inflammatory drug therapy. Arthritis Rheum. 1993; 36:84–90.
88. Piper DW, McIntosh JH, Ariotti DE, Fenton BH, MacLennan R. Analgesic ingestion and chronic peptic ulcer. Gastroenterology. 1981;80:427–32.
89. Rampton DS, McNeil NI, Sarner M. Analgesic ingestion and other factors preceding relapse in ulcerative colitis. Gut. 1983;24:187–9.
90. Flower RJ. Drugs which inhibit prostaglandin biosynthesis. Pharmacol Rev. 1974;26:33–67.
91. Robert A. Cytoprotection by prostaglandins. Gastroenterology. 1979;77:761–9.

24
The right time for medical or surgical treatment

D. MEYER and M. BÜTER

In order to find the right time for medical or surgical treatment you may use the following guidelines published by different societies, although even these guidelines do not give a clear answer to the subject:

1. *ASCRS (American Society of Colon and Rectal Surgeons)*. After two attacks of uncomplicated diverticulitis resection is recommended due to an increased risk of recurrent symptoms (7–45%) and lower expectancy of response to medical therapy (first attack 70%, third attack 6%)[1,2].

2. *Ad-hoc Practice Parameters (Committee of the American College of Gastroenterology)*. Most authorities agree that elective resection is indicated after two attacks of uncomplicated diverticulitis because recurrent attacks are less likely to respond to medical therapy and have a higher mortality rate[3].

3. *EAES Consensus Statement (European Association of Endoscopic Surgery)*. Patients should be considered for elective surgery if they have had at least two attacks of symptomatic diverticular disease. Surgery may also be indicated after the first attack in patients who require chronic immunosuppression. Chronic complications such as colovesicular or colovaginal fistulas, stenoses and bleeding are further indications for operation[4].

The authors agree that the second attack is the *turning point* for a decision between medical and surgical treatment. This is based on Parks' analysis from 1969, in which 455 patients with diverticular disease were observed retrospectively[5]. This study demonstrates a dramatic drop of response to medical treatment after the second episode. In contrast, Haglund observed in 392 patients with diverticular disease no difference in response to conservative treatment[6]. Due to their retrospective characters both studies have only a 3b evidence level. Unfortunately no prospective study is available for the natural history of diverticular disease. The question as to whether recurrent episodes of diverticular disease respond differently to antibiotics and parenteral therapy has been answered by two other studies (evidence level 3b): Makela et al.[7]

demonstrate on 366 retrospectively analysed patients that complications after the second episode increase up to 30%. In addition, Kaiser et al.[8] showed on 511 cases that failure from non-operative management correlates with the evidence of diverticular abscesses. Therefore, the following conclusion can be drawn: lower response rates to medical therapy after recurrent attacks are caused by an increased complication rate, mainly due to intra-abdominal or pelvic abscesses. These could not be observed by Parks because computed tomography (CT) technology was not routinely used in 1969. Uncomplicated episodes of diverticulitis respond even after the third episode to conservative treatment. Considering the increasing risk for complications, an individual decision should be made as to whether these patients need conservative therapy or a surgical resection of the diseased colon. This is confirmed in the guidelines of the American College of Gastroenterology (ASCRS) and the European Association of Endoscopic Surgery (EAES)[9]. They conclude that every patient needs an individual risk/benefit analysis, in which surgical therapy approaches are individualized for each patient and consideration is given to: (a) the severity and responsiveness of the attack, (b) general health of the patient, and (c) the risk for the patient of a subsequent attack.

Literature tells us that the risk for recurrence after second episodes is about 15–30%[10]. The mortality rate for elective surgery is 0–10%, for emergency surgery 15–30%. This should be discussed with the patient in order to discuss the right time for resection.

There are numerous retrospective studies which analyse the special history of diverticular disease in the young. However, the review by S. Janes, published in 2005 in the *British Journal of Surgery*, demonstrates that diverticular disease is not more violent in young patients, and surgical therapy is associated with a minimal mortality[11]. In conclusion, younger patients do not need more aggressive therapy. Therefore, the guidelines mentioned above can also be followed for young patients.

How should complications of diverticular disease such as bleeding, abscesses, fistulas or stenoses be treated?

1. *Bleeding*: most diverticular bleedings cease spontaneously, but a colonoscopy can be done in order to identify the course of lower gastrointestinal bleeding. In a case of recurrent haemorrhage, resection should be discussed in a semi-elective situation.

2. *Perforation/abscesses*: clinical symptoms and CT scan guide to a stage-related therapy. Pericolic or distant abscesses should be drained during CT study, which gives the opportunity for surgical resections of the diseased colon in a semi-elective situation. However, if clinical symptoms of peritonitis occur, and perforation or abscesses are demonstrated in the CT scan, an emergency operation is adequate.

3. *Fistula and stenoses*: both these complications of diverticular disease need surgery. This surgical treatment should be done in an elective situation to prevent a stoma, temporary or definitive (Hartmann procedure).

To summarize, the right time for medical or surgical treatment should be found in an individualized risk–benefit analysis. Lower responsiveness to medical treatment is due to increased complication rates after recurrent attacks. Development of complications represents a clear indication for surgery, but resection of the diseased colon should – if possible – be done in an elective or semi-elective situation, to prevent a Hartmann procedure. However, the mortality rate in both elective and emergency situations has been reduced when comparing the studies of the past 10 years. The hypothesis that younger patients should be treated more aggressively, due to their higher life expectancy and increased risk for recurrent attacks, cannot be confirmed, even though all studies on diverticular disease are done retrospectively only (evidence level 3).

References

1. Roberts P, Abel M, Rosen L, Cirocco W, Fleshman J, Leff EI. Standards Task Force, American Society of Colon and Rectal Surgeons. Practice parameters for sigmoid diverticulitis. Dis Colon Rectum. 1995;38:126–32.
2. Wong WD, Wexner SD, Lowry A et al. Practice parameters for the treatment of sigmoid diverticulitis – supporting documentation. Standards Task Force, American Society of Colon and Rectal Surgeons. Dis Colon Rectum. 2000;43: 290–7.
3. Stollman NH, Raskin JB. Diagnosis and management of diverticular disease of the colon in adults. Ad Hoc Practice Parameters Committee of the American College of Gastroenterology. Am J Gastroenterol. 1999;94:3110–21.
4. Kohler L, Sauerland S, Neugebauer E. Diagnosis and treatment of diverticular disease: results of a consensus development conference. Scientific Committee of the European Association for Endoscopic Surgery. Surg Endosc. 1999;13:430–6.
5. Parks TG. Natural history of diverticular disease of the colon. A review of 521 cases. Br Med J. 1969;4:639–42.
6. Haglund U, Hellberg R, Johnsen C, Hulten L. Complicated diverticular disease of the sigmoid colon. An analysis of short and long term outcome in 392 patients. Ann Chir Gynaecol. 1979;68:41–6.
7. Makela J, Vuolio S, Kiviniemi H, Laitinen S. Natural history of diverticular disease: when to operate? Dis Colon Rectum. 1998;41:1523–8.
8. Kaiser AM, Jiang JK, Lake JP et al. The management of complicated diverticulitis and the role of computed tomography. Am J Gastroenterol. 2005;100:910–17.
9. Stollman N, Raskin JB. Diverticular disease of the colon. Lancet. 2004;21:631–9.
10. Bokey EL, Chapius PH, Pheils MT. Elective resection for diverticular disease and carcinoma. Comparison of postoperative morbidity and mortality. Dis Colon Rectum. 1981;24:181–2.
11. Janes S, Meagher A, Frizelle FA. Elective surgery after acute diverticulitis. Br J Surg. 2005;92:133–42.

Index

Falk Symposium Series

43. Reutter W, Popper H, Arias IM, Heinrich PC, Keppler D, Landmann L, eds.: *Modulation of Liver Cell Expression.* Falk Symposium No. 43. 1987 ISBN: 0-85200-677-2*
44. Boyer JL, Bianchi L, eds.: *Liver Cirrhosis.* Falk Symposium No. 44. 1987 ISBN: 0-85200-993-3*
45. Paumgartner G, Stiehl A, Gerok W, eds.: *Bile Acids and the Liver.* Falk Symposium No. 45. 1987 ISBN: 0-85200-675-6*
46. Goebell H, Peskar BM, Malchow H, eds.: *Inflammatory Bowel Diseases – Basic Research & Clinical Implications.* Falk Symposium No. 46. 1988 ISBN: 0-7462-0067-6*
47. Bianchi L, Holt P, James OFW, Butler RN, eds.: *Aging in Liver and Gastrointestinal Tract.* Falk Symposium No. 47. 1988 ISBN: 0-7462-0066-8*
48. Heilmann C, ed.: *Calcium-Dependent Processes in the Liver.* Falk Symposium No. 48. 1988 ISBN: 0-7462-0075-7*
50. Singer MV, Goebell H, eds.: *Nerves and the Gastrointestinal Tract.* Falk Symposium No. 50. 1989 ISBN: 0-7462-0114-1
51. Bannasch P, Keppler D, Weber G, eds.: *Liver Cell Carcinoma.* Falk Symposium No. 51. 1989 ISBN: 0-7462-0111-7
52. Paumgartner G, Stiehl A, Gerok W, eds.: *Trends in Bile Acid Research.* Falk Symposium No. 52. 1989 ISBN: 0-7462-0112-5
53. Paumgartner G, Stiehl A, Barbara L, Roda E, eds.: *Strategies for the Treatment of Hepatobiliary Diseases.* Falk Symposium No. 53. 1990 ISBN: 0-7923-8903-4
54. Bianchi L, Gerok W, Maier K-P, Deinhardt F, eds.: *Infectious Diseases of the Liver.* Falk Symposium No. 54. 1990 ISBN: 0-7923-8902-6
55. Falk Symposium No. 55 not published

55B. Hadziselimovic F, Herzog B, Bürgin-Wolff A, eds.: *Inflammatory Bowel Disease and Coeliac Disease in Children.* International Falk Symposium. 1990 ISBN 0-7462-0125-7

56. Williams CN, eds.: *Trends in Inflammatory Bowel Disease Therapy.* Falk Symposium No. 56. 1990 ISBN: 0-7923-8952-2
57. Bock KW, Gerok W, Matern S, Schmid R, eds.: *Hepatic Metabolism and Disposition of Endo- and Xenobiotics.* Falk Symposium No. 57. 1991 ISBN: 0-7923-8953-0
58. Paumgartner G, Stiehl A, Gerok W, eds.: *Bile Acids as Therapeutic Agents: From Basic Science to Clinical Practice.* Falk Symposium No. 58. 1991 ISBN: 0-7923-8954-9
59. Halter F, Garner A, Tytgat GNJ, eds.: *Mechanisms of Peptic Ulcer Healing.* Falk Symposium No. 59. 1991 ISBN: 0-7923-8955-7
60. Goebell H, Ewe K, Malchow H, Koelbel Ch, eds.: *Inflammatory Bowel Diseases – Progress in Basic Research and Clinical Implications.* Falk Symposium No. 60. 1991 ISBN: 0-7923-8956-5
61. Falk Symposium No. 61 not published
62. Dowling RH, Folsch UR, Löser Ch, eds.: *Polyamines in the Gastrointestinal Tract.* Falk Symposium No. 62. 1992 ISBN: 0-7923-8976-X
63. Lentze MJ, Reichen J, eds.: *Paediatric Cholestasis: Novel Approaches to Treatment.* Falk Symposium No. 63. 1992 ISBN: 0-7923-8977-8
64. Demling L, Frühmorgen P, eds.: *Non-Neoplastic Diseases of the Anorectum.* Falk Symposium No. 64. 1992 ISBN: 0-7923-8979-4

64B. Gressner AM, Ramadori G, eds.: *Molecular and Cell Biology of Liver Fibrogenesis.* International Falk Symposium. 1992 ISBN: 0-7923-8980-8

*These titles were published under the MTP Press imprint.

Falk Symposium Series

65. Hadziselimovic F, Herzog B, eds.: *Inflammatory Bowel Diseases and Morbus Hirschprung*. Falk Symposium No. 65. 1992 ISBN: 0-7923-8995-6
66. Martin F, McLeod RS, Sutherland LR, Williams CN, eds.: *Trends in Inflammatory Bowel Disease Therapy.* Falk Symposium No. 66. 1993 ISBN: 0-7923-8827-5
67. Schölmerich J, Kruis W, Goebell H, Hohenberger W, Gross V, eds.: *Inflammatory Bowel Diseases – Pathophysiology as Basis of Treatment.* Falk Symposium No. 67. 1993 ISBN: 0-7923-8996-4
68. Paumgartner G, Stiehl A, Gerok W, eds.: *Bile Acids and The Hepatobiliary System: From Basic Science to Clinical Practice.* Falk Symposium No. 68. 1993 ISBN: 0-7923-8829-1
69. Schmid R, Bianchi L, Gerok W, Maier K-P, eds.: *Extrahepatic Manifestations in Liver Diseases.* Falk Symposium No. 69. 1993 ISBN: 0-7923-8821-6
70. Meyer zum Büschenfelde K-H, Hoofnagle J, Manns M, eds.: *Immunology and Liver.* Falk Symposium No. 70. 1993 ISBN: 0-7923-8830-5
71. Surrenti C, Casini A, Milani S, Pinzani M , eds.: *Fat-Storing Cells and Liver Fibrosis.* Falk Symposium No. 71. 1994 ISBN: 0-7923-8842-9
72. Rachmilewitz D, ed.: *Inflammatory Bowel Diseases – 1994*. Falk Symposium No. 72. 1994 ISBN: 0-7923-8845-3
73. Binder HJ, Cummings J, Soergel KH, eds.: *Short Chain Fatty Acids.* Falk Symposium No. 73. 1994 ISBN: 0-7923-8849-6

73B. Möllmann HW, May B, eds.: *Glucocorticoid Therapy in Chronic Inflammatory Bowel Disease: from basic principles to rational therapy.* International Falk Workshop. 1996 ISBN 0-7923-8708-2

74. Keppler D, Jungermann K, eds.: *Transport in the Liver.* Falk Symposium No. 74. 1994 ISBN: 0-7923-8858-5

74B. Stange EF, ed.: *Chronic Inflammatory Bowel Disease.* Falk Symposium. 1995 ISBN: 0-7923-8876-3

75. van Berge Henegouwen GP, van Hoek B, De Groote J, Matern S, Stockbrügger RW, eds.: *Cholestatic Liver Diseases: New Strategies for Prevention and Treatment of Hepatobiliary and Cholestatic Liver Diseases.* Falk Symposium 75. 1994. ISBN: 0-7923-8867-4
76. Monteiro E, Tavarela Veloso F, eds.: *Inflammatory Bowel Diseases: New Insights into Mechanisms of Inflammation and Challenges in Diagnosis and Treatment.* Falk Symposium 76. 1995. ISBN 0-7923-8884-4
77. Singer MV, Ziegler R, Rohr G, eds.: *Gastrointestinal Tract and Endocrine System.* Falk Symposium 77. 1995. ISBN 0-7923-8877-1
78. Decker K, Gerok W, Andus T, Gross V, eds.: *Cytokines and the Liver.* Falk Symposium 78. 1995. ISBN 0-7923-8878-X
79. Holstege A, Schölmerich J, Hahn EG, eds.: *Portal Hypertension.* Falk Symposium 79. 1995. ISBN 0-7923-8879-8
80. Hofmann AF, Paumgartner G, Stiehl A, eds.: *Bile Acids in Gastroenterology: Basic and Clinical Aspects.* Falk Symposium 80. 1995 ISBN 0-7923-8880-1
81. Riecken EO, Stallmach A, Zeitz M, Heise W, eds.: *Malignancy and Chronic Inflammation in the Gastrointestinal Tract – New Concepts.* Falk Symposium 81. 1995 ISBN 0-7923-8889-5
82. Fleig WE, ed.: *Inflammatory Bowel Diseases: New Developments and Standards.* Falk Symposium 82. 1995 ISBN 0-7923-8890-6

82B. Paumgartner G, Beuers U, eds.: *Bile Acids in Liver Diseases.* International Falk Workshop. 1995 ISBN 0-7923-8891-7

Falk Symposium Series

83. Dobrilla G, Felder M, de Pretis G, eds.: *Advances in Hepatobiliary and Pancreatic Diseases: Special Clinical Topics.* Falk Symposium 83. 1995. ISBN 0-7923-8892-5
84. Fromm H, Leuschner U, eds.: *Bile Acids – Cholestasis – Gallstones: Advances in Basic and Clinical Bile Acid Research.* Falk Symposium 84. 1995 ISBN 0-7923-8893-3
85. Tytgat GNJ, Bartelsman JFWM, van Deventer SJH, eds.: *Inflammatory Bowel Diseases.* Falk Symposium 85. 1995 ISBN 0-7923-8894-1
86. Berg PA, Leuschner U, eds.: *Bile Acids and Immunology.* Falk Symposium 86. 1996 ISBN 0-7923-8700-7
87. Schmid R, Bianchi L, Blum HE, Gerok W, Maier KP, Stalder GA, eds.: *Acute and Chronic Liver Diseases: Molecular Biology and Clinics.* Falk Symposium 87. 1996 ISBN 0-7923-8701-5
88. Blum HE, Wu GY, Wu CH, eds.: *Molecular Diagnosis and Gene Therapy.* Falk Symposium 88. 1996 ISBN 0-7923-8702-3

88B. Poupon RE, Reichen J, eds.: *Surrogate Markers to Assess Efficacy of TReatment in Chronic Liver Diseases.* International Falk Workshop. 1996 ISBN 0-7923-8705-8

89. Reyes HB, Leuschner U, Arias IM, eds.: *Pregnancy, Sex Hormones and the Liver.* Falk Symposium 89. 1996 ISBN 0-7923-8704-X

89B. Broelsch CE, Burdelski M, Rogiers X, eds.: *Cholestatic Liver Diseases in Children and Adults.* International Falk Workshop. 1996 ISBN 0-7923-8710-4

90. Lam S-K, Paumgartner P, Wang B, eds.: *Update on Hepatobiliary Diseases 1996.* Falk Symposium 90. 1996 ISBN 0-7923-8715-5
91. Hadziselimovic F, Herzog B, eds.: *Inflammatory Bowel Diseases and Chronic Recurrent Abdominal Pain.* Falk Symposium 91. 1996 ISBN 0-7923-8722-8

91B. Alvaro D, Benedetti A, Strazzabosco M, eds.: *Vanishing Bile Duct Syndrome – Pathophysiology and Treatment.* International Falk Workshop. 1996 ISBN 0-7923-8721-X

92. Gerok W, Loginov AS, Pokrowskij VI, eds.: *New Trends in Hepatology 1996.* Falk Symposium 92. 1997 ISBN 0-7923-8723-6
93. Paumgartner G, Stiehl A, Gerok W, eds.: *Bile Acids in Hepatobiliary Diseases – Basic Research and Clinical Application.* Falk Symposium 93. 1997 ISBN 0-7923-8725-2
94. Halter F, Winton D, Wright NA, eds.: *The Gut as a Model in Cell and Molecular Biology.* Falk Symposium 94. 1997 ISBN 0-7923-8726-0

94B. Kruse-Jarres JD, Schölmerich J, eds.: *Zinc and Diseases of the Digestive Tract.* International Falk Workshop. 1997 ISBN 0-7923-8724-4

95. Ewe K, Eckardt VF, Enck P, eds.: *Constipation and Anorectal Insufficiency.* Falk Symposium 95. 1997 ISBN 0-7923-8727-9
96. Andus T, Goebell H, Layer P, Schölmerich J, eds.: *Inflammatory Bowel Disease – from Bench to Bedside.* Falk Symposium 96. 1997 ISBN 0-7923-8728-7
97. Campieri M, Bianchi-Porro G, Fiocchi C, Schölmerich J, eds. *Clinical Challenges in Inflammatory Bowel Diseases: Diagnosis, Prognosis and Treatment.* Falk Symposium 97. 1998 ISBN 0-7923-8733-3
98. Lembcke B, Kruis W, Sartor RB, eds. *Systemic Manifestations of IBD: The Pending Challenge for Subtle Diagnosis and Treatment.* Falk Symposium 98. 1998 ISBN 0-7923-8734-1
99. Goebell H, Holtmann G, Talley NJ, eds. *Functional Dyspepsia and Irritable Bowel Syndrome: Concepts and Controversies.* Falk Symposium 99. 1998 ISBN 0-7923-8735-X
100. Blum HE, Bode Ch, Bode JCh, Sartor RB, eds. *Gut and the Liver.* Falk Symposium 100. 1998 ISBN 0-7923-8736-8

Falk Symposium Series

101. Rachmilewitz D, ed. *V International Symposium on Inflammatory Bowel Diseases.* Falk Symposium 101. 1998 ISBN 0-7923-8743-0
102. Manns MP, Boyer JL, Jansen PLM, Reichen J, eds. *Cholestatic Liver Diseases.* Falk Symposium 102. 1998 ISBN 0-7923-8746-5
102B. Manns MP, Chapman RW, Stiehl A, Wiesner R, eds. *Primary Sclerosing Cholangitis.* International Falk Workshop. 1998. ISBN 0-7923-8745-7
103. Häussinger D, Jungermann K, eds. *Liver and Nervous System.* Falk Symposium 102. 1998 ISBN 0-7924-8742-2
103B. Häussinger D, Heinrich PC, eds. *Signalling in the Liver.* International Falk Workshop. 1998 ISBN 0-7923-8744-9
103C. Fleig W, ed. *Normal and Malignant Liver Cell Growth.* International Falk Workshop. 1998 ISBN 0-7923-8748-1
104. Stallmach A, Zeitz M, Strober W, MacDonald TT, Lochs H, eds. *Induction and Modulation of Gastrointestinal Inflammation.* Falk Symposium 104. 1998 ISBN 0-7923-8747-3
105. Emmrich J, Liebe S, Stange EF, eds. *Innovative Concepts in Inflammatory Bowel Diseases.* Falk Symposium 105. 1999 ISBN 0-7923-8749-X
106. Rutgeerts P, Colombel J-F, Hanauer SB, Schölmerich J, Tytgat GNJ, van Gossum A, eds. *Advances in Inflammatory Bowel Diseases.* Falk Symposium 106. 1999 ISBN 0-7923-8750-3
107. Špičák J, Boyer J, Gilat T, Kotrlik K, Marećek Z, Paumgartner G, eds. *Diseases of the Liver and the Bile Ducts – New Aspects and Clinical Implications.* Falk Symposium 107. 1999 ISBN 0-7923-8751-1
108. Paumgartner G, Stiehl A, Gerok W, Keppler D, Leuschner U, eds. *Bile Acids and Cholestasis.* Falk Symposium 108. 1999 ISBN 0-7923-8752-X
109. Schmiegel W, Schölmerich J, eds. *Colorectal Cancer – Molecular Mechanisms, Premalignant State and its Prevention.* Falk Symposium 109. 1999 ISBN 0-7923-8753-8
110. Domschke W, Stoll R, Brasitus TA, Kagnoff MF, eds. *Intestinal Mucosa and its Diseases – Pathophysiology and Clinics.* Falk Symposium 110. 1999 ISBN 0-7923-8754-6
110B. Northfield TC, Ahmed HA, Jazwari RP, Zentler-Munro PL, eds. *Bile Acids in Hepatobiliary Disease.* Falk Workshop. 2000 ISBN 0-7923-8755-4
111. Rogler G, Kullmann F, Rutgeerts P, Sartor RB, Schölmerich J, eds. *IBD at the End of its First Century.* Falk Symposium 111. 2000 ISBN 0-7923-8756-2
112. Krammer HJ, Singer MV, eds. *Neurogastroenterology: From the Basics to the Clinics.* Falk Symposium 112. 2000 ISBN 0-7923-8757-0
113. Andus T, Rogler G, Schlottmann K, Frick E, Adler G, Schmiegel W, Zeitz M, Schölmerich J, eds. *Cytokines and Cell Homeostasis in the Gastrointestinal Tract.* Falk Symposium 113. 2000 ISBN 0-7923-8758-9
114. Manns MP, Paumgartner G, Leuschner U, eds. *Immunology and Liver.* Falk Symposium 114. 2000 ISBN 0-7923-8759-7
115. Boyer JL, Blum HE, Maier K-P, Sauerbruch T, Stalder GA, eds. *Liver Cirrhosis and its Development.* Falk Symposium 115. 2000 ISBN 0-7923-8760-0
116. Riemann JF, Neuhaus H, eds. *Interventional Endoscopy in Hepatology.* Falk Symposium 116. 2000 ISBN 0-7923-8761-9
116A. Dienes HP, Schirmacher P, Brechot C, Okuda K, eds. *Chronic Hepatitis: New Concepts of Pathogenesis, Diagnosis and Treatment.* Falk Workshop. 2000 ISBN 0-7923-8763-5

Falk Symposium Series

117. Gerbes AL, Beuers U, Jüngst D, Pape GR, Sackmann M, Sauerbruch T, eds. *Hepatology 2000 – Symposium in Honour of Gustav Paumgartner.* Falk Symposium 117. 2000 ISBN 0-7923-8765-1
117A. Acalovschi M, Paumgartner G, eds. *Hepatobiliary Diseases: Cholestasis and Gallstones.* Falk Workshop. 2000 ISBN 0-7923-8770-8
118. Frühmorgen P, Bruch H-P, eds. *Non-Neoplastic Diseases of the Anorectum.* Falk Symposium 118. 2001 ISBN 0-7923-8766-X
119. Fellermann K, Jewell DP, Sandborn WJ, Schölmerich J, Stange EF, eds. *Immunosuppression in Inflammatory Bowel Diseases – Standards, New Developments, Future Trends.* Falk Symposium 119. 2001 ISBN 0-7923-8767-8
120. van Berge Henegouwen GP, Keppler D, Leuschner U, Paumgartner G, Stiehl A, eds. *Biology of Bile Acids in Health and Disease.* Falk Symposium 120. 2001 ISBN 0-7923-8768-6
121. Leuschner U, James OFW, Dancygier H, eds. *Steatohepatitis (NASH and ASH).* Falk Symposium 121. 2001 ISBN 0-7923-8769-4
121A. Matern S, Boyer JL, Keppler D, Meier-Abt PJ, eds. *Hepatobiliary Transport: From Bench to Bedside.* Falk Workshop. 2001 ISBN 0-7923-8771-6
122. Campieri M, Fiocchi C, Hanauer SB, Jewell DP, Rachmilewitz R, Schölmerich J, eds. *Inflammatory Bowel Disease – A Clinical Case Approach to Pathophysiology, Diagnosis, and Treatment.* Falk Symposium 122. 2002 ISBN 0-7923-8772-4
123. Rachmilewitz D, Modigliani R, Podolsky DK, Sachar DB, Tozun N, eds. *VI International Symposium on Inflammatory Bowel Diseases.* Falk Symposium 123. 2002 ISBN 0-7923-8773-2
124. Hagenmüller F, Manns MP, Musmann H-G, Riemann JF, eds. *Medical Imaging in Gastroenterology and Hepatology.* Falk Symposium 124. 2002 ISBN 0-7923-8774-0
125. Gressner AM, Heinrich PC, Matern S, eds. *Cytokines in Liver Injury and Repair.* Falk Symposium 125. 2002 ISBN 0-7923-8775-9
126. Gupta S, Jansen PLM, Klempnauer J, Manns MP, eds. *Hepatocyte Transplantation.* Falk Symposium 126. 2002 ISBN 0-7923-8776-7
127. Hadziselimovic F, ed. *Autoimmune Diseases in Paediatric Gastroenterology.* Falk Symposium 127. 2002 ISBN 0-7923-8778-3
127A. Berr F, Bruix J, Hauss J, Wands J, Wittekind Ch, eds. *Malignant Liver Tumours: Basic Concepts and Clinical Management.* Falk Workshop. 2002 ISBN 0-7923-8779-1
128. Scheppach W, Scheurlen M, eds. *Exogenous Factors in Colonic Carcinogenesis.* Falk Symposium 128. 2002 ISBN 0-7923-8780-5
129. Paumgartner G, Keppler D, Leuschner U, Stiehl A, eds. *Bile Acids: From Genomics to Disease and Therapy.* Falk Symposium 129. 2002 ISBN 0-7923-8781-3
129A. Leuschner U, Berg PA, Holtmeier J, eds. *Bile Acids and Pregnancy.* Falk Workshop. 2002 ISBN 0-7923-8782-1
130. Holtmann G, Talley NJ, eds. *Gastrointestinal Inflammation and Disturbed Gut Function: The Challenge of New Concepts.* Falk Symposium 130. 2003 ISBN 0-7923-8783-X
131. Herfarth H, Feagan BJ, Folsch UR, Schölmerich J, Vatn MH, Zeitz M, eds. *Targets of Treatment in Chronic Inflammatory Bowel Diseases.* Falk Symposium 131. 2003 ISBN 0-7923-8784-8
132. Galle PR, Gerken G, Schmidt WE, Wiedenmann B, eds. *Disease Progression and Carcinogenesis in the Gastrointestinal Tract.* Falk Symposium 132. 2003 ISBN 0-7923-8785-6

Falk Symposium Series

132A. Staritz M, Adler G, Knuth A, Schmiegel W, Schmoll H-J, eds. *Side-effects of Chemotherapy on the Gastrointestinal Tract.* Falk Workshop. 2003 ISBN 0-7923-8791-0

132B. Reutter W, Schuppan D, Tauber R, Zeitz M, eds. *Cell Adhesion Molecules in Health and Disease.* Falk Workshop. 2003 ISBN 0-7923-8786-4

133. Duchmann R, Blumberg R, Neurath M, Schölmerich J, Strober W, Zeitz M. *Mechanisms of Intestinal Inflammation: Implications for Therapeutic Intervention in IBD.* Falk Symposium 133. 2004 ISBN 0-7923-8787-2

134. Dignass A, Lochs H, Stange E. *Trends and Controversies in IBD – Evidence-Based Approach or Individual Management?* Falk Symposium 134. 2004 ISBN 0-7923-8788-0

134A. Dignass A, Gross HJ, Buhr V, James OFW. *Topical Steroids in Gastroenterology and Hepatology.* Falk Workshop. 2004 ISBN 0-7923-8789-9

135. Lukáš M, Manns MP, Špičák J, Stange EF, eds. *Immunological Diseases of Liver and Gut.* Falk Symposium 135. 2004 ISBN 0-7923-8792-9

136. Leuschner U, Broomé U, Stiehl A, eds. *Cholestatic Liver Diseases: Therapeutic Options and Perspectives.* Falk Symposium 136. 2004 ISBN 0-7923-8793-7

137. Blum HE, Maier KP, Rodés J, Sauerbruch T, eds. *Liver Diseases: Advances in Treatment and Prevention.* Falk Symposium 137. 2004 ISBN 0-7923-8794-5

138. Blum HE, Manns MP, eds. *State of the Art of Hepatology: Molecular and Cell Biology.* Falk Symposium 138. 2004 ISBN 0-7923-8795-3

138A. Hayashi N, Manns MP, eds. *Prevention of Progression in Chronic Liver Disease: An Update on SNMC (Stronger Neo-Minophagen C).* Falk Workshop. 2004 ISBN 0-7923-8796-1

139. Adler G, Blum HE, Fuchs M, Stange EF, eds. *Gallstones: Pathogenesis and Treatment.* Falk Symposium 139. 2004 ISBN 0-7923-8798-8

140. Colombel J-F, Gasché C, Schölmerich J, Vucelic C, eds. *Inflammatory Bowel Disease: Translation from Basic Research to Clinical Practice.* Falk Symposium 140. 2005. ISBN 1-4020-2847-4

141. Paumgartner G, Keppler D, Leuschner U, Stiehl A, eds. *Bile Acid Biology and its Therapeutic Implications.* Falk Symposium 141. 2005 ISBN 1-4020-2893-8

142. Dienes H-P, Leuschner U, Lohse AW, Manns MP, eds. *Autoimmune Liver Disease.* Falk Symposium 142. 2005 ISBN 1-4020-2894-6

143. Ammann RW, Büchler MW, Adler G, DiMagno EP, Sarner M, eds. *Pancreatitis: Advances in Pathobiology, Diagnosis and Treatment.* Falk Symposium 143. 2005 ISBN 1-4020-2895-4

144. Adler G, Blum AL, Blum HE, Leuschner U, Manns MP, Mössner J, Sartor RB, Schölmerich J, eds. *Gastroenterology Yesterday – Today – Tomorrow: A Review and Preview.* Falk Symposium 144. 2005 ISBN 1-4020-2896-2

145. Henne-Bruns D, Buttenschön K, Fuchs M, Lohse AW, eds. *Artificial Liver Support.* Falk Symposium 145. 2005 ISBN 1-4020-3239-0

146. Blumberg RS, Gangl A, Manns MP, Tilg H, Zeitz M, eds. *Gut–Liver Interactions: Basic and Clinical Concepts.* Falk Symposium 146. 2005 ISBN 1-4020-4143-8

147. Jewell DP, Colombel JF, Peña AS, Tromm A, Warren BS, eds. *Colitis: Diagnosis and Therapeutic Strategies.* Falk Symposium 147. 2006 ISBN 1-4020-4315-5

148. Kruis W, Forbes A, Jauch K-W, Kreis ME, Wexner SD, eds. *Diverticular Disease: Emerging Evidence in a Common Condition.* Falk Symposium 148. 2006 ISBN 1-4020- 4317-1

MIX
Papier aus verantwortungsvollen Quellen
Paper from responsible sources
FSC® C105338

If you have any concerns about our products,
you can contact us on
ProductSafety@springernature.com

In case Publisher is established outside the EU,
the EU authorized representative is:
Springer Nature Customer Service Center GmbH
Europaplatz 3, 69115 Heidelberg, Germany

Printed by Libri Plureos GmbH
in Hamburg, Germany